The Right Imaging Study

A Guide for Physicians

Third Edition

The Right Imaging Study

A Guide for Physicians

Third Edition

Ronald L. Eisenberg, MD, JD
*Associate Professor of Radiology, Harvard
Medical School, Boston, Massachusetts, USA
Radiologist, Beth Israel Deaconess Medical
Center, Boston, Massachusetts, USA*

Alexander R. Margulis, MD
*Professor Emeritus, University of California at
San Francisco; Clinical Professor, Weill-Cornell Medical
College of Cornell University, New York, New York, USA*

With a Foreword by Robert B. Taylor, MD

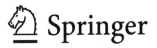 Springer

Editors
Ronald L. Eisenberg, MD, JD
Associate Professor of Radiology
Harvard Medical School
Boston, Massachusetts 02215
Radiologist,
Beth Israel Deaconess Medical Center
Boston, Massachusetts 02215

Alexander R. Margulis, MD
Professor Emeritus
University of California at San Francisco
Clinical Professor
Weill-Cornell Medical College of Cornell University
New York, New York 10065

ISBN: 978-0-387-73773-7   e-ISBN: 978-0-387-73774-4
DOI: 10.1007/978-0-387-73774-4

Library of Congress Control Number: 2007938315

The first and second editions of this book were published in 1996 and 2000,
respectively, by Lippincott Williams & Wilkins, Philadelphia, PA., with the
title *What to Order When: Pocket Guide to Diagnostic Imaging*.

Printed on acid-free paper

9 8 7 6 5 4 3 2 1

springer.com

To Zina, Avlana, and Cherina
and
To Hedi

Foreword

By Robert B. Taylor

In an ideal world, the process of obtaining and interpreting an imaging study for a patient would be true consultation between two specialists: The clinician who has examined the patient and who has primary responsibility for the patient's care would consult with a radiologist, and together they would select the most appropriate modality from among the panoply of imaging options available today.

Unfortunately, we live in an imperfect world, and such specialist-to-specialist consultation occurs all too infrequently. Instead, today the clinician is—in most instances—expected to know what diagnostic imaging study to order. With the time constraints and complexity of today's practice, what should be a consultation becomes an "order."

I am a family physician who has been in practice for more than four decades. Even with my long experience, I am sometimes not sure of the best imaging test to order for some patients. Perhaps you also have occasional questions you would like to ask a radiologist before ordering a study. For example: What modality is the "gold standard" for the noninvasive diagnosis of appendicitis? (It is computed tomography.) Can mammography detect saline implant rupture in the breast? (Yes, in all cases.) When might I order the Waters view of the paranasal sinuses? (It is useful for monitoring the treatment of acute sinusitis.) What is the role of radionuclide bone scanning in the diagnosis of osteomyelitis? (Little value.) And what is the most sensitive technique for detecting cerebral lesions responsible for headache? (It is magnetic resonance imaging. But patients with severe *acute* headaches should be imaged with noncontrast head CT because of the suspicion of subarachnoid hemorrhage, acute hydrocephalus, or an enlarging intracranial mass.)

Features of the book that appeal to me include the following: The book discusses what imaging studies may help elucidate the causes of everyday problems, such as diarrhea and dysuria, as well as more uncommon clinical entities, such as sarcoidosis and Reiter's syndrome. The likely causes of many signs and symptoms are listed, helping to guide the selection of the best study for the patient. Throughout the book are *Caveats,* such as: "Once the diagnosis of benign peptic ulcer disease has been made, recurrences should be treated symptomatically; there is no need to repeat an imaging procedure with each recurrence."

The book's outline format eliminates unnecessary verbiage, and in many instances the authors identify the "most effective" procedures and the "modality of choice." Appendix I describes the various imaging modalities available, and Appendix II tells the relative costs of these modalities to the patient, relative to the cost of a two-view chest radiograph. For example, the technical and professional fee to the patient for an MRI study is 8–12 times the cost of a routine chest x-ray.

And so, because most clinicians do not have a direct line and quick access to a radiologist, this book will be useful to the nonradiologists. In reviewing the manuscript, I found that it answered the questions above—and many more. In a sense, the book is like having a radiologic consultant "at your fingertips," and I think you will find it handy when deciding on the right imaging study. Keep the book in the location—probably your exam room—you are likely to be when deciding on imaging modalities to order, and perhaps have an extra copy for the staff person who actually schedules imaging studies.

Robert B. Taylor
Department of Family Medicine
Oregon Health and Science University
School of Medicine
Portland, Oregon

Preface to the Third Edition

In the last three decades, medical imaging has undergone tremendous advances, changing from a valuable diagnostic adjunct to an essential tool for diagnosis, selection of the optimal therapeutic approach, and treatment follow-up. It is now common practice that specialists summoned by emergency room staff will not see a patient before cross-sectional imaging procedures have been obtained and interpreted.

Important technological advances span the entire spectrum of imaging procedures. In MRI, new sequences increase speed and offer better definition. Increases in detector rows have made CT a three-dimensional modality and significantly improved its spatial resolution. In ultrasound, Doppler and harmonic imaging and the development of better contrast media have increased the information provided. Hybrid approaches to imaging are also rapidly emerging. PET/CT has become essential in oncology and is the first clinical approach of molecular imaging. PET/MRI will probably be coming soon. The combination of ultrasound and MRI will likely be employed for image-guided biopsies. MR spectroscopic imaging has become a valuable clinical tool in the evaluation of brain tumors and is being increasingly used in addition to MR in imaging cancer of the prostate.

Film as a recording device, like the flat plate at the dawn of radiology, has practically disappeared and been totally replaced by electronic digital records. PACS is ubiquitous, allowing communication between hospital departments, private offices, and even centers in different geographic locations. This technology has led to the development of teleradiography, with "nighthawk" services now available between different continents.

The dramatic advances in medical imaging have also produced some significant problems. The total cost of health care services in the USA has risen to 1.8 trillion dollars in 2006, exceeding 16% of the GNP. Although medical imaging is only a small part of these huge expenditures, it is now its most rapidly escalating segment. Consequently, requesting the right imaging procedure and avoiding a cascade of increasingly costly steps is essential in reducing costs.

The benefits derived from interventional radiology and CT are indisputable, but they are also adding to the ionizing radiation burden of the population. Therefore, being aware of the radiation exposure in requesting imaging studies is important. In addition, the increasing sophistication of the available imaging approaches makes it critical for the referring clinician to choose the right one to most expeditiously arrive at the diagnosis. These are among the compelling reasons for undertaking the writing of this book and enlisting the most prominent subspecialists in diagnostic imaging to collaborate.

The Right Imaging Study is designed to provide valuable assistance to residents-in-training and practicing physicians in internal medicine, general practice, emergency medicine, and surgery, as well as to other health care workers who are on the firing lines and actually request imaging studies. It is essential that these individuals have a clear understanding of the advantages and limitations of both newer and traditional imaging procedures, as well as their relative costs and ionizing radiation doses, so that they can make informed decisions regarding the most appropriate imaging strategies for their patients.

We are grateful to Dr. Robert Taylor, a prominent clinician who generously agreed to review the book from the standpoint of someone requesting imaging examinations and who also wrote the Foreword.

We hope that this book provides the information you need to best serve your patients.

Ronald L. Eisenberg
Alexander R. Margulis

Preface to the Second Edition

The format and approach of the first edition of this handbook has met our goal of providing a user-friendly guide to the most efficient and cost-effective imaging strategies for 300 clinical problems. Since its publication, managed care has become more prevalent and cost controls on medical care more stringent. With this in mind, the second edition offers updated imaging approaches (and some additional clinical situations) that reflect the continued technological advances in diagnostic imaging. For example, conventional radiography has become increasingly digital, with PACS making retrieval of images virtually instantaneous. In ultrasound, contrast media are now available, and harmonic imaging can diminish noise. Helical and multidetector CT have greatly improved patient throughput, and the reduction in price of nonionic contrast media has made their widespread use more feasible. Automation of reformatting has increased specificity and improved treatment planning. Single-shot sequencing has made MRI applicable in imaging the acute abdomen, while diffusion MR imaging is now available for diagnosing stroke at an early stage. Proton MR spectroscopy shows promise in the staging and treatment follow-up of prostate cancer and in evaluating brain tumors.

One further important change in the second edition is the new title, *What to Order When: Pocket Guide to Diagnostic*

Imaging. This change recognizes that a major audience for this book consists of residents-in-training and practicing physicians in internal medicine, general practice, emergency medicine, and surgery, and others who are on the firing lines and actually order imaging studies. It is essential that these physicians have a clear understanding of the advantages and limitations of both newer and traditional imaging procedures, as well as their relative costs, so that they can make informed decisions regarding the appropriate imaging strategies for their patients.

Medical imaging is rapidly advancing, and this pocket guide is designed to update physicians on the critical decision of *What to Order When*. In this way, physicians can ensure that their patients have the most appropriate imaging procedures that will lead to prompt diagnosis and timely treatment.

Ronald L. Eisenberg
Alexander R. Magulis

Preface to the First Edition

Medical imaging has made spectacular advances in the last 15 years, reflecting the explosive developments in computers, electronics, and television. New cross-sectional imaging modalities are now widely used for diagnosing a broad spectrum of clinical disorders. Ultrasound is the most available and least expensive of these new techniques, but it is highly operator-dependent and requires rigorous training of technologists and physicians. Computed tomography is extremely versatile and has better signal-to-noise ratios than ultrasound. However, it is more expensive, uses ionizing radiation, and often requires the use of iodinated contrast media. Magnetic resonance imaging is the most sophisticated of these cross-sectional techniques, offering the best soft-tissue contrast resolution and the ability to image directly in multiple planes with a variety of pulse sequences. However, it is the most expensive and time-consuming of these imaging modalities. Nuclear medicine procedures now provide metabolic as well as morphological information, especially when using highly sophisticated tomographic procedures (SPECT, PET). The major disadvantage of nuclear procedures is the need for the handling and disposal, the administration to patients, and in the case of PET, the very high cost of radioactive materials.

The availability of a wide variety of alternative imaging approaches comes at a time when the medical profession is facing severe financial constraints. Thus, it is essential that the practicing physician and resident-in-training have an understanding of the advantages and limitations of the newer (and the traditional) imaging procedures and a conception of their relative costs.

To meet this critical need, we have developed the *Radiology Pocket Reference* to recommend the most efficient and cost-effective imaging strategies for 300 clinical problems. The book is organized to reflect the two basic situations that the clinician faces when ordering an image study. The first part of each section deals with those symptoms and signs that do not permit a single working diagnosis. The second part provides coherent strategies that can be used when there is a working clinical diagnosis to be confirmed, refined, or rejected by imaging procedures. For every symptom or sign, a list of differential diagnoses is offered; for each clinical diagnosis, there is a brief outline of typical signs and symptoms as well as predisposing factors.

Our guiding principle in selecting the order of imaging examinations has been the need to combine cost effectiveness and noninvasiveness with high diagnostic accuracy. However, the reader must always take into consideration such local conditions as the availability and adequacy of equipment and the expertise of the radiologists performing the recommended studies. Therefore, we often suggest alternative approaches to be taken when modern equipment and adequate expertise are not available.

To fit the goal of a pocket-sized book that would receive frequent use, we have used a terse outline approach, choosing to include more clinical scenarios at the expense of long explanations. We intentionally did not burden the reader with detailed statistical information on sensitivity, specificity, accuracy, and positive and negative predictive values, because these figures vary greatly, are often in dispute, and are constantly changing. Similarly, we chose not to include specific references that would have made the book substantially longer without providing any additional practical information. Nevertheless, we have taken a wealth of experimental data into account in selecting those procedures that provide the highest likelihood of leading to the diagnosis.

To ensure that the information provided to the reader is up to date, each chapter has been edited by a prominent radiologist subspecializing in that area (in most instances the author of a highly regarded textbook in the field). Rather than repeat the same information throughout the book, we have included an appendix that describes the basics of each of the newer sophisticated imaging modalities as well as the relative costs of individual procedures in multiples of the basic chest radiograph.

We sincerely hope that the pocket-sized format of the book will make it readily available when it is needed most—in the many clinical situations in which there is not enough time to go to the medical library and consult larger, more encyclopedic texts. We intend to keep this reference book current by adding or deleting information as it becomes available in the literature. To meet our overall goal, we would appreciate receiving suggestions from readers concerning ways in which we could make this pocket-sized reference book even more user-friendly.

Ronald L. Eisenberg
Alexander R. Margulis

Contents

Contributors

Daniel Brewer, M.D.
Associate Professor, Department of Family Medicine,
University of Tennessee Medical Center, University of
Tennessee, Knoxville, Knoxville, Tennessee, USA

D. David Dershaw, M.D.
Director, Breast Imaging Section, Department of
Radiology, Memorial Sloan-Kettering Cancer Center,
New York, New York, USA

William Dillon, M.D.
Professor of Radiology, Neurology, and Neurosurgery,
University of California School of Medicine,
San Francisco, California, USA

Burton P. Drayer, M.D.
Charles and Marilyn Newman Professor and Chair,
Department of Radiology, The Mount Sinai Medical
Center, New York, New York, USA

N. Reed Dunnick, M.D.
Fred Jenner Hodges Professor and Chair, Department of
Radiology, University of Michigan, Ann Arbor, Michigan,
USA

Richard M. Gore, M.D.
Professor of Radiology, Department of Radiology,
Northwestern University Medical School, Chicago,
Illinois, USA
and
Chief, Section of Gastrointestinal Radiology, Evanston
Hospital—McGaw Medical Center of Northwestern
University, Evanston, Illinois, USA

Hedvig Hricak, M.D.
Chairman, Department of Radiology, Memorial
Sloan-Kettering Cancer Center, New York, New York, USA

Jeffrey S. Klein, M.D.
A. Bradley Seule and John P. Tampas Green and Gold
Professor of Radiology, Department of Radiology,
University of Vermont College of Medicine, Burlington,
Vermont, USA

Deborah Levine, M.D.
Associate Radiologist-in-Chief of Academic Affairs,
Co-Chief of Ultrasound, Director of Obstetrics/Gynecology
Ultrasound, Department of Radiology, Beth Israel
Deaconess Medical Center, Harvard Medical School,
Boston, Massachusetts, USA

Donald Resnick, M.D.
Professor of Radiology, University of California,
San Diego, La Jolla, California, USA
and
Chief, Osteoradiology Section, Veterans Administration
Medical Center, San Diego, California, USA

Evis Sala, M.D.
University Lecturer, Department of Radiology, University
of Cambridge, Addenbrooke's Hospital, Cambridge, UK

U. Joseph Schoepf, M.D.
Associate Professor of Radiology and Medicine,
Department of Radiology, Medical University of South
Carolina, Charleston, South Carolina, USA

1

NECK AND FACE
William Dillon

Thyroid Mass

Common Causes

Diffuse or nodular goiter
Thyroiditis
Abscess
Cyst
Neoplasm (adenoma, carcinoma, metastases, lymphoma)

Approach to Diagnostic Imaging

Note: In most centers, the diagnostic work-up for a solitary thyroid nodule no longer includes radionuclide thyroid scanning.

■ 1. Radionuclide thyroid scan

- May differentiate hypofunctioning (cold) nodules (10–20% representing carcinoma) and hyperfunctioning (hot) nodules (5–8% malignant)

 Caveat: Although radionuclide scan can detect thyroid nodules, it cannot discriminate benign from malignant processes.

■ 2. Ultrasound

- Primarily indicated to determine whether a non-functioning thyroid mass detected on a radio-nuclide scan is cystic or solid (purely cystic or hyperechoic masses are rarely malignant) and whether there are single or multiple nodules
- Of special value in patients in whom exogenous iodine contamination from prior contrast studies precludes a radionuclide scan
- Perhaps its most important role is in guiding fine needle aspiration for cytologic analysis

 Caveat: As with radionuclide scan, US cannot determine whether a hypoechoic mass is benign or malignant.

■ 3. Magnetic resonance imaging

- Useful in defining the extent of thyroid neoplasms

Note: CT and MRI are primarily used to demonstrate a substernal thyroid that cannot be detected by US because of overlying bone.

■ 4. Fine needle aspiration biopsy (FNAB)

- FNAB has emerged as the most important step in the diagnostic evaluation of thyroid nodules. A highly accurate procedure, in experienced hands FNAB has a mean sensitivity and a mean specificity of >80% and >90%, respectively. FNAB can reduce the need for diagnostic thyroidectomy by 20–50% and increase the yield of cancer diagnoses in thyroid specimens by 15–45%.

Neck Mass

Presenting Signs and Symptoms

Enlarging neck mass, either in or off the midline
Usually painless, unless secondary to infection

Common Causes

PRIMARY

Midline mass
  Thyroglossal duct cysts
  Dermoid/epidermoid cysts
Paramedian neck mass
  Branchial cleft cyst
  Cystic hygroma (cavernous lymphangioma)
  Neuroma (rare)

SECONDARY

Cervical adenopathy (usually metastatic from head
  and neck primary)
Cervical adenitis and abscess (signs of infection)

Approach to Diagnostic Imaging

■ 1. Computed tomography

- Thin-section (<3 mm) helical CT with contrast is
  the best modality for demonstrating the extent
  of disease

■ 2. Magnetic resonance imaging

- Preferred modality for evaluating mucosal surfaces
  in patients with suspected carcinoma of the aero-
  digestive tract (T1- and T2-weighted sequences,
  fat-saturation images with contrast)
- Sagittal imaging is useful for delineating the cranial–caudal dimension of thyroglossal duct cysts

Hypercalcemia

Presenting Signs and Symptoms

Usually asymptomatic (discovered incidentally during routine laboratory screening)

Constipation, anorexia, nausea and vomiting, abdominal pain, adynamic ileus

Nephrolithiasis (or urolithiasis) and nephrocalcinosis; polyuria, nocturia, and polydipsia; renal failure

Skeletal muscular weakness

Emotional lability, confusion, delirium, psychosis, stupor, coma

Common Causes

Hyperparathyroidism (primary)

Chronic renal failure (secondary hyperparathyroidism)

Excessive gastrointestinal absorption and/or intake (milk-alkali syndrome, vitamin D intoxication, sarcoidosis)

Endocrine dysfunction (hypothyroidism, Addison's disease)

Skeletal metastases, multiple myeloma

Humoral hypercalcemia of malignancy (no bone metastases)

Immobilization

Drug therapy (thiazides, lithium, aluminum-containing antacids)

Approach to Diagnostic Imaging

Clinical assessment is necessary to direct the imaging approach

Radiographs of the hands, pelvis, and spine are useful for evaluating hyperparathyroidism (hands) or metastasis or myeloma (pelvis, spine)

Note: See individual underlying disorders.

Hyperparathyroidism

Presenting Signs and Symptoms

May be asymptomatic (50%)
Renal disease (nephrolithiasis and nephrocalcinosis)
Peripheral neuromuscular disease (proximal muscle weakness, fatiguability, atrophy)
Gastrointestinal disease (peptic ulcers, pancreatitis)
Neuropsychiatric dysfunction

Common Causes

PRIMARY

Parathyroid adenoma (89%)
Parathyroid hyperplasia (10%)
Parathyroid carcinoma (1%)

SECONDARY

Chronic renal failure

Paraneoplastic Syndromes

Bronchogenic carcinoma
Renal cell carcinoma

Approach to Diagnostic Imaging

- **1. Plain skeletal radiograph (hands, other skeletal sites)**
  - May demonstrate characteristic:
    - Subperiosteal resorption of radial aspect of the middle phalanges of the hand
    - Resorption of phalangeal tufts
    - Erosion of distal clavicles
    - Sclerotic stripes in vertebral bodies ("rugger jersey" spine)
    - Punched-out lesions in the skull ("salt-and-pepper" appearance)

> **Note:** Although once routinely obtained, there is no need for a "metabolic bone survey" (including the long bones and spine), because the yield of positive findings is extremely low and a positive finding rarely affects treatment. If any radiographic study is required, plain films of the hands should suffice.

Detection of Parathyroid Gland Abnormality

■ 1. Ultrasound

- Detects 80–85% of abnormal parathyroid glands located near the thyroid
- Most important use is guiding fine needle aspiration biopsy for cytology
- Parathyroid carcinomas tend to have a more heterogeneous internal architecture than adenomas

■ 2. Computed tomography or magnetic resonance imaging

- Generally required to detect abnormal parathyroid tissue at ectopic sites such as the thymus (10–15%), the posterior mediastinum (5%), the carotid sheath, and the retroesophageal or parapharyngeal region

■ 3. Radionuclide dual phase technetium imaging (Technetium 99m-sestamibi [Tc99m-MIBI])

- Detects parathyroid adenomas and hyperplasia (sensitivity 83%; 75% specificity) and is more sensitive than ultrasound (sensitivity 65%). The combination of this technique with ultrasound improves sensitivity and specificity.

Hyperthyroidism

Presenting Signs and Symptoms

Goiter
Weight loss with increased appetite
Warm, moist skin
Heat intolerance
Tremor
Irritability and insomnia
Palpitations and tachycardia
Muscle weakness
Exophthalmos
Frequent bowel movements
Thyroid storm (thyrotoxicosis)
Proptosis

Common Causes

Graves' disease (toxic diffuse goiter)
Toxic multinodular goiter (Plummer's disease)
Toxic adenoma
Thyroiditis (subacute or painless)
Thyrotoxicosis factitia (ingestion of thyroid hormone tablets)

Approach to Diagnostic Imaging

Caveat: The diagnosis of hyperthyroidism is made clinically by routine thyroid hormone determinations, and there usually is no need for routine imaging studies.

■ 1. Radionuclide thyroid scan (either I-123 or technetium-99m)

- Indicated if the etiology of hyperthyroidism is not clear after physical examination and laboratory testing
- Can distinguish Graves' disease from multinodular goiter or a single toxic adenoma

■ 2. Radioactive iodine uptake

- Although long used to measure thyroid function, this test has been supplanted by radioimmunoassay techniques and the development of accurate methods to measure serum levels of thyroid hormones and stimulating factors
- I-123 iodine uptake scintigraphy is currently performed primarily for differentiating Graves' disease (high uptake) from subacute or painless thyroiditis (low uptake), and in assisting in the calculation of the dose of radioactive iodine required for the treatment of Graves' disease

■ 3. Computed tomography (orbits)

- May be required in the diagnosis of Graves' ophthalmopathy, in which diffuse enlargement of the extraocular muscles results in proptosis, chemosis, and occasionally visual loss from compression of the optic nerve

Hypothyroidism (Myxedema)

Presenting Signs and Symptoms

Weight gain
Dull facial expression with hoarse voice and slow speech
Periorbital swelling and drooping eyelids
Cold intolerance
Sluggishness
Sparse, coarse, dry hair
Coarse, dry, scaly skin
Constipation

Common Causes

Dietary iodine deficiency (endemic goiter)
Chronic thyroiditis (Hashimoto's disease)
Treated hyperthyroidism (radioactive iodine or surgery)
Failure of hypothalamic–pituitary axis (deficient secretion of thyrotropin-releasing hormone or thyroid-stimulating hormone)

Approach to Diagnostic Imaging

Caveat: The diagnosis of hypothyroidism is made clinically by routine thyroid hormone determinations, and there usually is no need for routine imaging studies.

Note: Although long used to measure thyroid function, radionuclide iodine uptake has been supplanted by radioimmunoassay techniques and the development of accurate methods to measure serum levels of thyroid hormones and stimulating factors.

Cancer of the Larynx

Presenting Signs and Symptoms

Neck mass (cervical adenopathy) in a smoker older than age 40 (men more often than women)
Hoarseness
Stridor

Common Sites

True vocal cord
Supraglottic soft tissues

Approach to Diagnostic Imaging

■ 1. Computed tomography

- Thin-section CT is the best modality for demonstrating the extent of tumor and the presence of cervical adenopathy

■ 2. Magnetic resonance imaging

- Preferred modality for evaluating the mucosa and cartilage involvement
- Superior to CT for defining the infraglottic spread of disease

 Caveat: Because post-biopsy changes may simulate occult carcinoma, CT and MRI should be performed before biopsy, if possible.

Cancer of the Pharynx

Presenting Signs and Symptoms

Neck mass (cervical adenopathy) in a smoker older than age 40 (more often men than women)
Referred otalgia (ear pain)
Chronic sore throat or tongue ulceration
Cranial nerve palsy
Decreased hearing (due to serous effusion within the ear)

Common Sites

Tongue, floor of mouth, tonsil, oropharynx, base of tongue, pyriform sinus (nasopharynx is less common)

Approach to Diagnostic Imaging

■ 1. Magnetic resonance imaging

- Preferred modality for evaluating the pharyngeal mucosa and other sites where occult disease may reside
- Superior technique for defining intracranial spread of disease and involvement of the carotid artery

■ 2. Computed tomography

- Helical CT may permit evaluation of the site of the neck mass and cervical adenopathy

Note: On CT, contrast infusion is required to differentiate lymph nodes from vessels.

Caveat: Because post-biopsy changes may simulate occult carcinoma, CT and MRI should be performed before biopsy, if possible.

Cancer of the Thyroid

Presenting Signs and Symptoms

Asymptomatic (felt by the patient or detected on physical examination)

Recurrent laryngeal palsy

Hoarseness

Metastasis to cervical nodes or remote sites

Approach to Diagnostic Imaging

■ 1. Radionuclide thyroid scan

- Single hypofunctioning (cold) nodule has a 10–20% chance of being malignant

Note: A history of neck irradiation, especially in childhood, increases the risk of malignancy by 5–10 times.

■ 2. Ultrasound

- Primarily indicated to determine whether a nonfunctioning thyroid mass detected on a radionuclide scan is cystic or solid (purely cystic or hyperechoic masses are rarely malignant)
- Of special value in patients in whom exogenous iodine contamination from prior contrast studies precludes a radionuclide scan

 Caveat: Because neither radionuclide scan nor US (nor CT nor MRI) can definitely determine whether a nonfunctioning, hypoechoic mass is benign or malignant, aspiration biopsy is required in every suspicious case.

Note: Regression of nodule size following thyroid hormone therapy is a sign of a benign nodule.

Staging

■ 1. Computed tomography or magnetic resonance imaging

- Procedures of choice for demonstrating involvement of adjacent muscles, larynx, esophagus, and other neck structures by invasive tumor
- MRI may better demonstrate the relationship of the carotid vessels to the tumor; CT is easier for imaging the chest and mediastinum

■ 2. Whole-body radionuclide scan (iodine-131)

- Effectively demonstrates thyroid metastases following thyroidectomy for *papillary* carcinoma

 Caveat: This technique is of no value for medullary and anaplastic carcinomas because these tumors do not take up iodine.

■ 3. Positron emission tomography

- Most sensitive technique for the detection of cervical adenopathy, particularly in those patients with thyroid carcinoma who have negative I-131 scans.

Detecting Recurrences

■ 1. Magnetic resonance imaging

- Modality of choice for detecting recurrent tumor, which appears as an area of high signal intensity on T2-weighted images

> **Note:** On T2-weighted images, fibrosis has low signal intensity that is less than or equal to that of adjacent muscle.

■ 2. Whole-body radionuclide scan (iodine-131)

- Focal activity in the lungs, skeleton, or neck remote from the thyroid bed is evidence of recurrence

> **Note:** Uptake of radionuclide in the thyroid bed often represents residual thyroid tissue; uptake in the stomach, bowel, bladder, and salivary glands reflects physiologic traces of normal iodine distribution; and uptake in the breast also may be a normal finding.

■ 3. Positron emission tomography

- PET scanning with FDG is a sensitive diagnostic tool that can be used in patients with a known history of thyroid cancer, including those with elevated thyroglobulin. Unlike the use of I-131 for diagnosis, PET does not require the routine discontinuation of TSH suppression.

Salivary Gland (Parotid) Neoplasm

Presenting Signs and Symptoms

Palpable mass (slightly tender or nontender)

Facial palsy

Parapharyngeal mass

If *benign cyst,* tends to develop quickly over several days, may be tender if infected, and often has a history of prior recurrent episodes

If *benign tumor,* slow-growing, painless, nontender, and mobile

If *malignant tumor,* tends to enlarge rapidly over several weeks and be slightly painful and minimally tender, hard and fixed on palpation, and often associated with facial nerve paralysis

Approach to Diagnostic Imaging

■ 1. Computed tomography or magnetic resonance imaging

- Preferred studies for identifying:
  - Presence of a mass or multiple masses
  - Mass location within the gland and position relative to the facial nerve
  - Whether the mass is smoothly marginated or infiltrating and necrotic, or cystic or solid
  - Whether the mass is confined to the gland or has extended outside the gland capsule into the upper neck and skull base
  - CT is superior to MRI for detecting an underlying calcified stone (calculus)

- MRI is superior to CT for sharply outlining the margins of the mass (what CT shows as a vague fullness may appear as a discrete mass on MRI; or what CT shows as several different masses may be shown to be a highly lobulated solitary mass on MRI)

 Caveat: The distinction between a benign and a malignant mass often cannot be made purely on the basis of CT or MRI. However, when imaging findings are combined with clinical findings, an accuracy rate of about 90% can be achieved.

Note: Fine-needle biopsy, often performed under CT guidance, can provide a precise pathologic diagnosis in more than 90% of patients.

Occult Primary With Positive Lymphadenopathy

Presenting Sign and Symptom

Neck mass in a smoker older than age 40 (men more often than women)

Common Causes

Squamous carcinoma of the pharynx, tonsil, pyriform sinus, nasopharynx, or base of the tongue

Approach to Diagnostic Imaging

■ 1. Magnetic resonance imaging

- Preferred imaging modality for evaluating the pharyngeal mucosa and other sites where the occult malignancy may reside

■ 2. Computed tomography

- High-speed studies may detect the site of an occult carcinoma in about 25% of cases (thus permitting directed biopsy by endoscopy)

 Caveat: Because post-biopsy changes may simulate occult carcinoma, MRI and CT should be performed before biopsy, if possible.

■ 3. Positron emission tomography

- More sensitive than MR or CT in detecting the primary tumor in patients who present with cervical adenopathy

Internal Disk Derangement of Temporomandibular Joint

Presenting Signs and Symptoms

Clicking or popping sound when opening the mouth (anterior subluxation with reduction of the disk)

Painful limitation of jaw movement (anterior subluxation without reduction of the disk)

Common Causes

Chronic spasm of the lateral pterygoid muscle

Trauma

Arthritic changes in the temporomandibular joint

Approach to Diagnostic Imaging

■ 1. Magnetic resonance imaging

- Preferred modality for evaluating displacement of the disk and whether there is reduction during function (should be performed in the open- and closed-mouth positions with the use of surface coils)

Note: Arthrography and CT are not as effective as MRI for imaging internal disk derangements of the temporomandibular joint.

Cranial Neuropathy

Common Causes

Neoplasm (primary or perineural spread of existing tumor)
Infection (viral or bacterial)
Radiation therapy

Approach to Diagnostic Imaging

■ 1. Magnetic resonance imaging

- Study of choice for assessing cranial neuropathy of undetermined cause

Note: This study should be performed using contrast-enhanced, fat-saturated imaging perpendicular to the course of the affected cranial nerve.

 Caveat: MR scans must examine the entire course of the nerve from its origin in the brain stem to its distal ramifications.

■ 2. Computed tomography

- Less sensitive than MRI for detecting early spread of carcinoma along cranial nerves

Note: CT should be performed using thin sections oriented to the appropriate plane of section and perpendicular to the involved nerve.

Specific Cranial Nerves

TRIGEMINAL NEUROPATHY (NOT TIC DOULOUREUX)

Most commonly due to a cerebellopontine angle mass, schwannoma of the trigeminal nerve, or perineural spread of tumor from the oral cavity or the head and neck

FACIAL PALSY

Most common cause is Bell's palsy (viral neuritis)

Does not require imaging confirmation unless facial function is slow to return or there is some other complicating factor (pain, dysfunction of other cranial nerves, parotid mass)

Must exclude parotid malignancy and temporal bone tumors (hemangioma, cholesteatoma, neurinoma) as well as skull base infections (diabetics), brainstem lesions in children, and Lyme disease in patients living in endemic regions.

Trauma is a leading cause of facial palsy and requires CT in the proper clinical setting.

Note: MRI is the imaging study of choice for the brain stem and parotid gland; CT may be useful for evaluating the temporal bone.

LOWER CRANIAL NERVES (9–12)

Most commonly due to a tumor at the skull base, which is best demonstrated by MRI

Differential diagnosis includes paraganglioma, meningioma, metastasis, and primary skull base tumor (e.g., chondrosarcoma)

Vocal cord paralysis may be due to a lesion anywhere from the skull base down to the hila of the lung (CT is the optimal imaging study)

THIRD CRANIAL NERVE

Common causes include diabetes, infarction, and leptomeningeal disease such as metastatic tumor

In the setting of an unexplained third nerve palsy, MR angiography, CT angiography, or conventional arteriography is indicated to exclude an expanding aneurysm of the carotid or posterior communicating artery

Sinusitis

Presenting Signs and Symptoms

Pain, tenderness, and swelling over the involved sinus
Eye pain, fever, chills (suggesting extension of infection
   beyond the sinuses)

Predisposing Factors

Recent acute viral upper respiratory infection
Dental infection

Approach to Diagnostic Imaging

■ 1. Computed tomography

- Procedure of choice for exquisitely defining the
  sinonasal anatomy and infections of the paranasal sinuses and the soft tissues of the head
  and neck

Note: Both axial and coronal planes (direct imaging
or reformations) are suggested to detect sinusitis or
suspected complications of sinusitis such as mucocele
or osteomyelitis. However, CT findings often do not
correlate with the patient's clinical symptoms. Mild
mucosal thickening (<4mm) without an associated
fluid level is a nonspecific finding that is frequently
seen in asymptomatic individuals who undergo head
or orbital CT for other medical complaints, as well
as in patients with a common cold (upper respiratory
viral infection).

■ 2. Magnetic resonance imaging

- Indicated for suspected neoplasm, detection of intracranial spread of infection, or in patients with neurological symptoms
- May be the best modality for detecting and characterizing obstructive sinonasal secretions or mucocele
- Contrast MRI is the best technique for detecting subdural or epidural empyema

■ 3. Plain radiograph (sinus)

- Limited role in assessing sinus disease
- Waters view is useful for monitoring treatment of acute sinusitis

 Caveat: MRI should be restricted to assessing complications of sinusitis and should not be used as a screening examination.

Vocal Cord Paralysis

Presenting Signs and Symptoms

Unilateral or bilateral, complete or incomplete

Signs and symptoms relate to the underlying pathologic process, which often arises at some distance from the larynx

Common Causes

Chest lesions affecting the recurrent laryngeal nerve (e.g., bronchial or esophageal carcinoma, metastatic mediastinal nodes, pulmonary tuberculosis, aortic arch aneurysm, cardiac surgery)

Neck lesions affecting the recurrent laryngeal nerve (e.g., thyroid surgery, penetrating wound, malignant cervical nodes, carcinoma of the hypopharynx, thyroid, or esophagus)

Previous surgical procedure in the neck or chest

Lesion affecting the vagal nerve in the jugular foramen (nasopharyngeal carcinoma, schwannoma or paraganglioma of the jugular foramen, idiopathic)

Uncommon Cause

Brain stem lesions affecting vagal nerve nuclei in the medulla

Approach to Diagnostic Imaging

■ 1. Plain chest radiograph

- Initial procedure for excluding lung cancer or apical thoracic tuberculosis

■ 2. Barium swallow

- Indicated if there is clinical evidence of a primary esophageal cause

■ 3. Computed tomography

- Excellent imaging study for detecting any structural abnormality of the neck or chest affecting the recurrent laryngeal nerve
- Reformatted images may be particularly informative

■ 4. Magnetic resonance imaging

- Examination of choice if a brain stem or skull base etiology is suspected
- Ability to image in coronal and sagittal planes makes MRI superior to CT for detecting apical chest lesions
- May be better than CT for assessing the neck (due to high soft-tissue resolution)
- Complementary with CT in evaluating lesions in or near the skull base

Epiglottitis

Presenting Signs and Symptoms

Stridor
Difficulty swallowing, drooling
Rigid neck
High fever in acutely ill patient (typically ages 3–6)

Common Cause

Haemophilus influenzae type B infection

Approach to Diagnostic Imaging

■ 1. Plain lateral radiograph of the neck (soft-tissue technique)

- Preferred imaging technique for demonstrating characteristic enlargement of the epiglottis ("thumb sign") that narrows the airway

---

Note: There is *no* indication for any other imaging study. The thickness of the epiglottis is normally 3–5 mm; detection of an epiglottis that is ≥7 mm thick is 100% sensitive and specific for epiglottis.

2

CHEST

Jeffrey S. Klein

Acute Respiratory Failure

Common Causes

Chronic obstruction pulmonary disease (exacerbation)

Lower respiratory tract infection (pneumonia)

Central nervous system depression (head trauma or injudicious use of sedatives, narcotics, tranquilizers, or oxygen

Cardiovascular disorders (myocardial infarction, heart failure, pulmonary emboli)

Non-cardiogenic pulmonary edema (ARDS)

Airway irritants (smoke or fumes)

Acute asthma attack

Endocrine and metabolic disorders (myxedema, metabolic alkalosis)

Thoracic abnormalities (chest trauma, pneumothorax, thoracic or abdominal surgery)

Approach to Diagnostic Imaging

■ 1. Plain chest radiograph

- Preferred initial imaging technique to detect the spectrum of findings that can be produced by the numerous conditions that can cause acute respiratory failure

■ 2. Computed tomography

- Provides more specific information regarding parenchymal, pleural, and airway abnormalities that may produce acute respiratory failure (e.g., early ARDS, atypical pneumonia)

Cough

Common Causes

Inflammatory (laryngitis, tracheitis, bronchitis, bronchiolitis, bronchiectasis, pneumonia, lung abscess, asthma)

Mechanical (compression or compromise of airway due to neoplasm, foreign body, granulomas, bronchospasm)

Inhalation of particulate material (pneumoconioses)

Chemical (inhalation of irritant fumes, including cigarette smoke, gastroesophageal reflux)

Thermal (inhalation of cold or very hot air)

Medications (e.g., angiotensin converting enzyme inhibitors)

Approach to Diagnostic Imaging

■ 1. Plain chest radiograph

- Preferred imaging technique to demonstrate infection, neoplasm, or diffuse pulmonary parenchymal disease

Notes: Additional imaging studies are rarely needed, except for appropriate follow-up radiographs, because the overwhelming majority of patients with clinically significant new cough will have pneumonia, bronchitis, or some other acute infectious disease of the respiratory tract.

Because a negative chest radiograph does not exclude pneumonia (or cancer), especially in immunocompromised patients, if an antibiotic-sensitive infection is suspected clinically, a sputum specimen should be obtained and the patient treated despite the unrevealing film.

■ 2. Computed tomography

- Useful for detecting central airway lesions, particularly in patients at risk for bronchogenic carcinoma or who have hemoptysis

Cyanosis

Presenting Signs and Symptoms

Bluish discoloration of the skin or mucous membranes (due to excess of reduced hemoglobin in the blood)

Common Causes

Impaired pulmonary function (pneumonia, pulmonary edema, chronic obstructive pulmonary disease)

Anatomic vascular shunting (congenital heart disease, pulmonary arteriovenous malformation)

Decreased oxygen in inspired air (high altitude)

Abnormal hemoglobin

Approach to Diagnostic Imaging

■ 1. Plain chest radiograph

- Preferred imaging technique to demonstrate underlying pulmonary or cardiac abnormality

■ 2. Computed tomography

- To detect pulmonary disease as the cause of hypoxemia and cyanosis

■ 3. Echocardiography

- To detect right-to-left intracardiac or extracardiac shunts

■ 4. Magnetic resonance imaging

- For evaluation of cyanosis associated with congenital heart disease

Dyspnea (Shortness of Breath)

Presenting Signs and Symptoms

Shortness of breath
Difficulty breathing on exertion
Uncomfortable awareness of breathing (increased muscular
    effort required)

Common Causes

Physical exertion
Hypoxia (high altitude)
Restrictive lung disease (pulmonary fibrosis, chest wall
    deformity, pleural fibrosis)
Obstructive lung disease (emphysema, asthma)
Congestive heart failure
Pulmonary embolism

Approach to Diagnostic Imaging

■ 1. Plain chest radiograph

- Best imaging technique for identifying an underlying pulmonary or cardiac cause, as well as any
  need for appropriate additional imaging studies

> **Note:** Soft-tissue views of the neck (or fiberoptic
> examination) may be helpful in patients with suspected
> acute upper airway obstruction.

■ 2. Computed tomography

- Useful for evaluation of parenchymal lung disease,
  central airway compromise, and pulmonary
  embolism (contrast-enhanced) as causes of
  dyspnea

Hemoptysis

Presenting Signs and Symptoms

Coughing up blood (resulting from bleeding from the respiratory tract)

Common Causes

Infection (pneumonia, tuberculosis, fungal infection, lung abscess)
Bronchogenic carcinoma
Bronchiectasis
Bronchitis
Pulmonary infarction (secondary to embolism)
Congestive heart failure
Pulmonary hemorrhage syndromes (e.g., Goodpasture's syndrome, Wegener's granulomatosis)

Approach to Diagnostic Imaging

■ 1. Plain chest radiograph

- Initial imaging procedure
- Normal study does not exclude neoplasm or bronchiectasis as the cause of the bleeding

■ 2. Computed tomography

- Indicated in a patient with a normal chest radiograph in whom the clinical suspicion of malignancy is relatively low
- Indicated if a neoplasm is not detected by fiberoptic bronchoscopy (which is unreliable in locating peripheral tumors demonstrable by CT)
- Indicated in any patient with recurrent symptoms of bronchitis or bronchiectasis

 Caveat: Despite a systematic and intensive search, the cause of hemoptysis will not be found in 30–40% of patients.

■ 3. Fiberoptic bronchoscopy

- Indicated in a patient for whom there is a high clinical suspicion of malignancy and who has a relevant abnormality on the plain chest radiograph
- Relatively invasive procedure with potential complications (e.g., hemorrhage, pneumothorax, hypoxemia)

Pleuritic Pain

Presenting Signs and Symptoms

Pain that is aggravated by breathing or coughing (may be of sudden onset, chronic, or recurring)

Rapid and shallow respiration

Limited motion of the affected side

Decreased breath sounds on the affected side

Pleural friction rub (characteristic finding that is often absent and is frequently heard only 24–48 h after the onset of pain)

Common Causes

Pneumonia

Tuberculosis

Pulmonary embolism

Trauma

Neoplasm

Occult rib fracture

Congestive heart failure

Mixed connective tissue disease

Pancreatitis

Approach to Diagnostic Imaging

■ 1. Plain chest radiograph

- Preferred imaging technique that may demonstrate the underlying pulmonary, rib, or chest wall abnormality, as well as a confirming pleural effusion

■ 2. Computed tomography

- Useful for evaluating pleural disease, peripheral pleural-based parenchymal inflammatory or neoplastic processes, chest wall lesions or injury, and pulmonary embolism (contrast-enhanced) that may produce pleuritic chest pain

Stridor/Upper Airway Obstruction

Presenting Signs and Symptoms

Musical sound that is predominantly inspiratory and is loud enough to be heard without a stethoscope at some distance from the patient (heard better over the neck than over the chest)

Common Causes

Epiglottitis
Croup
Inhaled foreign body
Pharyngeal tumor
Glottic edema
Retropharyngeal abscess
Vocal cord dysfunction

Approach to Diagnostic Imaging

■ 1. Plain radiograph of the neck (soft-tissue technique)

- Preferred imaging technique to demonstrate narrowing or luminal obstruction of the upper airway (lateral projection is often more valuable than the frontal view)

> **Note:** Laryngoscopy or CT of the neck may be required, especially in older patients in whom malignancy is more common and infection is a less likely cause. Laryngoscopy is also necessary for a diagnosis of vocal cord dysfunction as a cause of stridor.

Wheezing

Presenting Signs and Symptoms

Wheezing or whistling noise associated with breathing
(implies obstruction to the flow of air at some level in
the respiratory tract)
Most commonly heard on expiration

Common Causes

Asthma
Congestive heart failure
Pneumonia
Bronchogenic tumor
Pulmonary embolus
Tracheobronchomalacia
Foreign body

Approach to Diagnostic Imaging

■ **1. Plain chest radiograph**

- Preferred imaging study to exclude a tumor or a foreign body

■ **2. Computed tomography**

- Preferred method to noninvasively evaluate the trachea and central airways for masses, narrowing, or compression that is not evident on plain chest radiographs. Dynamic expiratory CT with reduced radiation dose is useful for assessment of dynamic airway collapse in tracheobronchomalacia

Abstract (Lung)

Presenting Signs and Symptoms

Cough productive of moderate-to-large amounts of purulent, often foul-smelling sputum that may be tinged with blood

Fever and sweats

Chest pain and dyspnea

Anorexia and weight loss

Leukocytosis

Approach to Diagnostic Imaging

■ 1. Plain chest radiograph

- Preferred initial imaging technique to demonstrate an area of consolidation that may develop into a cavity with an air–fluid level after rupture of the abscess into the bronchial tree
- May permit differentiation of a peripheral lung abscess (round; formation of an acute angle with the chest wall) from an empyema (lenticular shape; formation of an obtuse angle with the chest wall)

■ 2. Computed tomography

- Best modality for differentiating peripheral lung abscess from empyema

---

Note: Most lung abscesses can be treated with antibiotic therapy and postural drainage; empyemas require a drainage procedure.

■ 3. Fiberoptic bronchoscopy

- May allow the removal of an underlying foreign body or excessive mucus and permit material to be obtained for culture
- Also useful in patients with suspected central airway masses producing postobstructive pneumonia/abscess

Adult Respiratory Distress Syndrome (ARDS)

Presenting Signs and Symptoms

Tachypnea, then dyspnea (24–48 h after initial illness/injury)

Noncardiogenic pulmonary edema

Hypoxemia and cyanosis

Common Causes

Diffuse pulmonary infection (bacterial or viral)

Aspiration of gastric contents

Direct chest trauma

Prolonged or profound shock

Inhalation of toxins and irritants

Systemic reaction to nonpulmonary processes (e.g., gram-negative septicemia, hemorrhagic pancreatitis, fat embolism)

Massive blood transfusion

Cardiopulmonary bypass ("pump lung")

Narcotic overdose pulmonary edema

Burns

Near-drowning

Acute upper airway obstruction

Approach to Diagnostic Imaging

■ 1. Plain chest radiograph

- Nonspecific diffuse bilateral opacities similar to pulmonary edema (but cardiac silhouette within normal size and no pleural effusion)
- Findings may lag many hours behind functional changes and appear much less severe than the clinical degree of hypoxemia
- Required during mechanical ventilation to detect evidence of barotrauma (pneumothorax, pneumomediastinum) and to evaluate tube placements (endotracheal, chest, and nasogastric tubes; Swan-Ganz catheter; central venous line)

■ 2. Computed tomography

- Often helps characterize parenchymal abnormalities in patients with ARDS and detects complications of mechanical ventilation

Asbestosis

Presenting Signs and Symptoms

Insidious onset of exertional dyspnea and reduced exercise tolerance

Symptoms of airways disease (cough, sputum, wheezing) occurring primarily in heavy smokers

Common Causes

Occupational exposure

Approach to Diagnostic Imaging

■ 1. Plain chest radiograph

- Preferred initial imaging technique to demonstrate irregular or linear small opacities (usually most prominent in the lower zones) and characteristic diffuse or localized pleural thickening (calcified or non-calcified pleural plaques)

- Relatively low specificity because of frequent difficulty in differentiating pleural thickening from normal intercostal muscles and extrapleural fat companion shadows of the chest wall (more likely asbestos-related if bilateral, symmetric, and along the midlateral chest wall)

■ 2. High-resolution computed tomography

- Superior to chest radiography for detecting pleural plaques
- Superior to chest radiography in detecting and characterizing patients with mild parenchymal changes not evident radiographically
- Not recommended as a screening examination because of its high cost (good-quality chest radiographs interpreted by an informed reader have a high sensitivity and negative predictive value in the diagnosis of pleural plaques)
- Valuable for eliminating false-positive diagnoses of noncalcified plaques caused by muscle or fat and for distinguishing pleural plaques from lung

Asthma

Presenting Signs and Symptoms

Episodic respiratory distress, often with tachypnea, tachycardia, and audible wheezes

Anxiety and struggling for air

Use of accessory muscles of respiration

Hyperexpansion of the lung (due to air trapping)

Prolonged expiratory phase

Approach to Diagnostic Imaging

■ 1. Plain chest radiograph

- Findings varying from entirely normal to hyper-inflation, increased lung opacities, bronchial wall thickening, and regions of atelectasis

 Caveat: Once the diagnosis of asthma is established, chest radiographs are only required during recurrent episodes when there is clinical suspicion of complications (e.g., pneumothorax, atelectasis, secondary infection).

■ 2. Fiberoptic bronchoscopy

- Indicated in a patient who has the potential for aspiration of a foreign body or is unresponsive to medical management. Also useful to diagnosis vocal cord dysfunction, which may mimic asthma clinically.

■ 3. Computed tomography

- Indicated in a patient with chronic bronchospasm when chest radiography is normal
- May reveal focal opacities of increased attenuation with air trapping (mosaic perfusion). This heterogeneous pattern could reflect bronchiolitis obliterans, hypersensitivity pneumonitis, or allergic alveolitis
- Can detect airway disease that may be mistaken for asthma clinically and not detected on plain chest radiographs (e.g., carcinoid tumor, bronchogenic carcinoma)

Atelectasis

Presenting Signs and Symptoms

Depend on the speed of the bronchial occlusion, the extent of lung affected, and the presence of infection

Common Causes

Mucous plugs (tenacious bronchial exudate)
Endobronchial tumor
Granuloma
Foreign body
Extrinsic compression of a bronchus (by enlarged lymph nodes, tumor, aneurysm)
Extrapulmonary external compression of the lung (pleural effusion, pneumothorax), which is termed passive atelectasis
Space-occupying intrapulmonary mass (e.g., bulla, large lung tumor), which is termed compressive atelectasis
Neonatal respiratory distress syndrome (decreased or abnormal surfactant)
Pulmonary embolism
Infection
Postoperative (diaphragmatic dysfunction, pain)
Postinflammatory scarring (cicatricial)

Approach to Diagnostic Imaging

■ 1. Plain chest radiograph

- Preferred imaging technique to demonstrate characteristic linear streaks (plate-like atelectasis) or a segment of shrunken, airless lung
- If atelectasis involves a substantial amount of the lung, the chest radiograph may show secondary elevation of the ipsilateral hemidiaphragm; shift of the trachea, heart, and mediastinum toward the affected area; and modification of the normal pulmonary vascular pattern
- May show the underlying cause of atelectasis (extrinsic mass, pleural effusion, pneumothorax)

■ 2. Fiberoptic bronchoscopy or computed tomography

- Indicated to search for a cause of obstruction if there is no other obvious source for a collapsed segment or lobe

Note: Fiberoptic bronchoscopy may be therapeutic as well as diagnostic (e.g., removal of mucous plugs, obtaining material for culture or cytology).

Bronchiectasis

Presenting Signs and Symptoms

Chronic cough with sputum production (often after severe
pneumonia with incomplete clearing of symptoms)
Hemoptysis
Recurrent pneumonia
Chronic atelectasis

Common Causes

Recurrent or chronic pneumonia
Chronic aspiration
Cystic fibrosis
Allergic bronchopulmonary aspergillosis
Interstitial pulmonary fibrosis
Tuberculous scarring (upper lobes)
Intrinsic bronchial disease (stenosis, extrinsic compression,
endobronchial mass)

Approach to Diagnostic Imaging

■ 1. Plain chest radiograph

- Abnormal in most patients, but the specific diagnosis can be suggested less than one-half the time
- Demonstrates increased interstitial opacities from
  recurrent inflammatory or infectious responses or
  changes consistent with subsegmental atelectasis
- Often "tram tracking" (parallel linear shadows
  representing the walls of cylindrically dilated
  bronchi) and areas of multiple thin-walled
  cysts, with or without air–fluid levels, which
  tend to be peripheral and cluster together in the
  distribution of a bronchovascular bundle

2. High-resolution computed tomography

- High accuracy for demonstrating characteristic multiple, dilated, thin-walled circular lucencies (on cross-section) and parallel linear opacities (bronchial walls sectioned lengthwise)
- Mucoid impactions may simulate lung nodules or branching, finger-like opacities
- Cystic bronchiectasis produces a "cluster of grapes" appearance
- Detection of central varicose bronchiectasis is highly suggestive of allergic bronchopulmonary aspergillosis
- May show evidence of inhomogeneous lung attenuation (mosaic perfusion), reflecting abnormal lung ventilation and resultant reduced perfusion

Note: CT has all but eliminated the need for contrast bronchography, except for those few patients considered for curative resection who appear to have localized disease according to CT.

3. Fiberoptic bronchoscopy

- While thin-section CT has become the mainstay modality in the evaluation of bronchiectasis, bronchoscopy may be useful for performing contrast bronchography in the assessment of focal bronchiectasis, particularly in patients under consideration for possible surgical resection
- Bronchoscopy also may be useful in excluding abnormalities associated with bronchiectasis, such as tumors, foreign bodies, and stenosis

Bronchogenic Carcinoma

Presenting Signs and Symptoms

Cough (with or without hemoptysis)
Dyspnea, wheezing, pneumonia
Chest pain
Weight loss
History of smoking
Pleural effusion
Recurrent Horner's syndrome
Superior vena cava syndrome
Symptoms relating to distal metastases (e.g., occult fracture, seizure)

Note: The lesion may be an asymptomatic pulmonary nodule discovered incidentally on a routine chest radiograph or chest computed tomography.

Risk Factors

Cigarette smoking
Occupational exposure (e. g., asbestos, radiation, arsenic, chromates, nickel, mustard gas, radon)
Pulmonary fibrosis (e.g., old inflammatory disease such as tuberculosis, or diffuse interstitial fibrosis as in idiopathic pulmonary fibrosis)

Approach to Diagnostic Imaging

■ 1. Plain chest radiograph

- Preferred initial imaging technique to demonstrate a solitary pulmonary nodule, atelectasis, pulmonary opacity, bronchial narrowing, hilar or mediastinal lymphadenopathy, or pleural effusion

■ 2. Computed tomography

- Permits percutaneous fine-needle biopsy of peripheral lesions to obtain material for cytologic studies

Staging

■ 1. Computed tomography (chest/upper abdomen) or PET/CT

- Definitive noninvasive study
- Detects hilar and mediastinal lymphadenopathy and bronchial narrowing
- May show metastases in the liver and adrenal glands

Note: MRI may be valuable for detecting vascular invasion and mediastinal spread of tumor, evaluating local extension of superior sulcus tumors into the brachial plexus, and for clarifying whether adrenal enlargement is due to metastases or a benign cause.

Bronchitis (Chronic)

Presenting Signs and Symptoms

Chronic productive cough (excessive tracheobronchial mucus secretion sufficient to cause cough with expectoration of sputum that occurs on most days for at least 3 consecutive months in at least 2 consecutive years)

Common Causes

Cigarette smoking
Occupational exposure
Air pollution and other types of bronchial irritation
Chronic pneumonia
Superimposed emphysema

Approach to Diagnostic Imaging

■ 1. Plain chest radiograph

- Normal examination in about one-half of patients
- May demonstrate nonspecific appearance with prominence of interstitial markings and thickened bronchial walls

---

Note: Chronic bronchitis is a clinical and not a radiographic diagnosis. Once the diagnosis of chronic bronchitis is established, chest radiographs are only required if there is clinical suspicion of a supervening acute pneumonia or a developing malignancy.

Bronchopleural Fistula

Presenting Signs and Symptoms

Fever, cough, dyspnea, pleurisy

Intractable pneumothorax

Large air leak in a person with a pleural drain

Common Causes

Dehiscence of bronchial stump after lobectomy or pneumonectomy

Necrotizing pulmonary infection

Carcinoma of the lung with pleural invasion

Approach to Diagnostic Imaging

■ 1. Plain chest radiograph

- ■ Demonstrates a loculated intrapleural collection of air and fluid (with an air–fluid level on upright films)

Note: In bronchopleural fistula, the air–fluid level has unequal dimensions on frontal and lateral radiographs due to its lenticular shape; this is in contrast to lung abscess, in which the dimension of the air–fluid level remains stable between frontal and lateral projections due to its round shape.

■ 2. Computed tomography

- Can often distinguish a bronchopleural fistula from a peripheral lung abscess
- Occasionally may demonstrate the actual fistulous communication
- Useful for planning external drainage of infected pleural collections resulting from a bronchopleural fistula

■ 3. Sinogram

- Injection of contrast material into a chest tube draining the pleural space may demonstrate the site of bronchial communication

Chest Tube/Line/Catheter Placement

Indication for Study

Determination of the tip of a radiopaque tube/line/catheter placed within the thorax

Detecting complications of line placement (i.e., pneumothorax, hemorrhage)

Common Types

Endotracheal tube
Central venous pressure (CVP) catheter
Dialysis catheter
Swan-Ganz catheter
Nasogastric tube
Mediastinal drain
Intra-aortic balloon pump
Pacemaker/implantable cardioverter-defibrillator

Approach to Diagnostic Imaging

■ 1. Plain chest radiograph

- Demonstrates whether the tip of the tube/line/catheter is in the proper position
- **Endotracheal tube:** With the head in a neutral position, the tip should be 5–7 cm above the carina

Note: With flexion and extension of the neck, the tip of the tube will move about 2 cm caudally and cranially, respectively.

- **CVP catheter:** Within the superior vena cava (above the level of the right atrium, to prevent irritation of the sinoatrial node and ectopic beats), preferably at the level of the carina

Note: Up to one-third of CVP catheters are incorrectly placed at the time of initial insertion.

- **Dialysis catheter:** Within the right atrium to ensure consistently good blood flow
- **Swan-Ganz catheter:** Within the right or left main pulmonary arteries

Note: Too peripheral a position of the tip may lead to occlusion of the pulmonary artery and resulting distal pulmonary infarction or insufflation injury to a peripheral pulmonary artery branch with pseudoaneurysm formation.

- **Nasogastric tube:** Stomach

Note: The tip of the tube may remain in the esophagus above the esophagogastric junction or be misplaced in the bronchial tree or into the pleural space.

- **Mediastinal drain:** Anteriorly positioned behind the sternum (occasionally beneath the heart and above the diaphragm)
- **Intra-aortic balloon pump:** Tip should be in the upper descending thoracic aorta, below the top of the knob (i.e., below the origin of the left subclavian artery)
- **Pacemaker:** Atrial lead should be in the right atrial appendage, right ventricular lead in the right ventricular apex, left ventricular lead in the coronary sinus/great cardiac vein (dual chamber pacemaker)

Emphysema

Presenting Signs and Symptoms

Exertional dyspnea (gradually progressive)
Productive cough
Abnormal pulmonary function tests

Common Causes

Cigarette smoking
Occupational exposure
α_1-antitrypsin deficiency
Congenital

Approach to Diagnostic Imaging

■ 1. Plain chest radiograph

- Lungs often appear normal in mild disease
- Eventually demonstrates hyperexpansion of the lungs (depressed diaphragm, generalized radiolucency of the lungs, enlarged retrosternal air space, ability to see diaphragmatic insertions from the lower ribs) and focal opacities due to atelectasis or scarring
- Bullous changes (especially in the apices and subpleural regions)
- Marked attenuation and stretching (even virtual absence) of pulmonary vessels
- Often evidence of pulmonary hypertension (enlargement of central pulmonary arteries with rapid peripheral tapering)
- In α_1-antitrypsin deficiency, emphysematous changes predominantly involve the lower lobes

Caveat: Once the diagnosis of emphysema is established, repeated chest radiographs are only indicated if there is clinical indication of supervening disease (e.g., infection, congestive heart failure).

■ 2. High-resolution computed tomography

- More sensitive than conventional radiography for detecting emphysematous changes in the lungs, but rarely necessary. (The extent of clinical derangement is generally determined by pulmonary function tests.)
- Of special value in detecting otherwise unsuspected blebs and bullae in select high-risk populations, such as those with suspected α_1-antitrypsin deficiency or with recurrent pneumothoraces
- May be of value in preoperative assessment of patients considered for lung volume reduction surgery as treatment of upper-lobe-predominant emphysema.

Empyema

Presenting Signs and Symptoms

Chest pain (varies from vague discomfort to stabbing pain and is often worse with coughing or breathing)
Rapid, shallow breathing
Fever, chills, night sweats
Cough
Weight loss

Note: If an empyema develops during the course of antibiotic treatment for bacterial pneumonia, the symptoms may be mild and the condition may go unrecognized.

Common Causes

Acute pneumonia
Lung abscess
Thoracic surgery or trauma
Spread from extrapulmonary sites (osteomyelitis of spine, subphrenic abscess)
Sepsis
Tuberculosis

Approach to Diagnostic Imaging

■ 1. Plain chest radiograph

- Preferred initial imaging technique
- May permit differentiation of empyema (lenticular shape; formation of an obtuse angle with the chest wall) from lung abscess (round; formation of an acute angle with the chest wall)

■ 2. Computed tomography

- Best modality for differentiating empyema from peripheral lung abscess

---

Note: Empyema requires a drainage procedure; most lung abscesses can be treated with antibiotic therapy and postural drainage.

- May show contrast enhancement of the parietal and visceral pleura, thickening of the extrapleural subcostal tissues, and increased attenuation of the extrapleural fat, which are rarely seen with transudative effusions

■ 3. Thoracentesis

- Required to confirm suspected empyema to avoid a delay in diagnosis, which may have serious consequences

■ 4. Ultrasound

- Can help confirm the presence of a parapneumonic effusion in a patient with pneumonia
- Can serve as a valuable guide for obtaining fluid from a loculated empyema

Eosinophilic Lung Disease

Presenting Signs and Symptoms

Range from mild respiratory symptoms and low fever (and prompt recovery) to severe pulmonary symptoms in a life-threatening condition

Striking blood eosinophilia (the exception is acute eosinophilic pneumonia)

Coexistent asthma

Common Causes

Drug-induced eosinophilic lung disease (penicillin, aminosalicylic acid, hydralazine, chlorpropamide, sulfonamides)

Hypersensitivity pneumonitis (extrinsic allergic alveolitis)

Asthmatic pulmonary eosinophilia (hypersensitivity bronchopulmonary aspergillosis)

Tropical eosinophilia (parasites such as roundworm, filaria)

Pulmonary eosinophilia (Löffler's syndrome)

Approach to Diagnostic Imaging

■ 1. Plain chest radiograph

- Preferred imaging technique for detecting the broad spectrum of pulmonary abnormalities seen in these disorders

■ 2. Computed tomography

- Infrequently required in a symptomatic patient with normal chest radiographs as a "road map" prior to biopsy and as an aid to following the response to treatment
- Classic peripheral, non-segmental consolidation in two thirds of patients with chronic eosinophilic pneumonia.

Hypersensitivity Lung Disease

Presenting Signs and Symptoms

Acute: Dyspnea, fever, chills

Subacute and chronic forms: Progressive cough, shortness of breath

Restrictive lung function with concomitant obstruction not uncommon

Serum precipitins sensitive but not specific for diagnosis

Common Causes

Farmer's lung (moldy hay)

Bird-fancier's lung (avian antigens)

Hot-tub lung (mycobacterium avium-intracellulare)

Approach to Diagnostic Imaging

■ 1. Plain chest radiograph

- Shows diffuse ground-glass or fine nodular or reticulonodular opacities (acute and subacute forms)
- Upper lobe reticulation, retraction with volume loss

■ 2. High-resolution computed tomography

- Ground-glass opacities (acute form)
- Centrilobular ground-glass nodules with an upper lobe predilection (subacute disease)
- Upper zone reticulation with traction bronchiectasis, honeycombing (chronic form)

Infectious Granulomatous Disease

Presenting Signs and Symptoms

Varies from asymptomatic exposure to fever, productive cough, and night sweats

Common Causes

Tuberculosis (especially in HIV-positive patients and in immigrants from Asia and Central America)

Histoplasmosis (central and eastern United States)

Coccidioidomycosis (southwestern United States and Mexico)

Blastomycosis (south-central and midwestern United States)

Cryptococcosis

Approach to Diagnostic Imaging

■ 1. Plain chest radiograph

- Preferred imaging technique to show the various patterns of opacifications within the lung (lobar consolidation, nodular opacities ranging from miliary to more discrete nodules, masses suggesting neoplasm, and diffuse disease with or without pleural effusion)
- Best imaging modality for identifying potential complications (empyema, extensive atelectasis, and focal or diffuse dissemination of the primary disease)

■ 2. High-resolution computed tomography

- Indicated if there are any questions concerning the findings on plain radiographs

Mediastinal Mass (Superior)

Presenting Signs and Symptoms

Asymptomatic and incidental finding on plain chest radiograph

Displacement, deviation, or compression of the trachea (upper thoracic portion)

Common Causes

Substernal thyroid

Lymph node enlargement

Parathyroid mass

Other causes of anterior, middle, or posterior mediastinal masses

Approach to Diagnostic Imaging

■ 1. Plain chest radiograph

- Detects a mass displacing, deviating, or compressing the trachea but otherwise does little to characterize the mass

■ 2. Radionuclide thyroid scan

- Most accurate method for diagnosing the presence of abnormal thyroid tissue in the neck or superior mediastinum

■ **3. Computed tomography**
- Definitive imaging study for defining the origin and extent of the mass and for determining its underlying characteristics

■ **4. Magnetic resonance imaging**
- Equivalent to CT in confirming the presence and location of a mediastinal mass
- Less effective than CT for assessing tracheal involvement and for demonstrating calcification
- Superior to CT for distinguishing tumor from fibrosis and in patients in whom the use of iodinated contrast material is contraindicated

Mediastinal Mass (Anterior)

Presenting Signs and Symptoms

Asymptomatic and incidental finding on plain chest radiograph

Myasthenia gravis (in up to 30–50% of patients with thymoma)

Cough, chest pain (local compression)

B symptoms with fever, sweats, weight loss (lymphoma)

Common Causes

Thymoma

Teratoma

Lymphoma

Parathyroid tumor (ectopic)

Aortic aneurysm (ascending portion)

Morgagni hernia

Approach to Diagnostic Imaging

■ 1. Plain chest radiograph

- Detects and determines precise compartment of a mediastinal mass but otherwise does little to characterize the mass (can rarely demonstrate specific findings, such as teeth within a mature teratoma or peripheral calcification within an aortic aneurysm)

■ 2. Computed tomography

- Definitive imaging study for defining the origin and extent of a mass and determining its underlying characteristics
- With contrast enhancement, highly accurate in differentiating among fatty, cystic, and soft-tissue masses and aneurysms
- Can aid in differential diagnosis by detecting calcification not evident on plain radiographs

■ 3. Magnetic resonance imaging

- Equivalent to CT in confirming the presence and location of a mediastinal mass
- Less effective than CT for assessing tracheal involvement and demonstrating calcification
- Superior to CT for distinguishing tumor from fibrosis and in patients in whom the use of iodinated contrast material is contraindicated

Mediastinal Mass (Middle)

Presenting Signs and Symptoms

Asymptomatic and incidental finding on plain chest radiograph

Compression of trachea or esophagus (dysphagia, stridor, cough, wheezing, or localized or diffuse chest pain—depends more on size of mass than on its identity)

Common Causes

Lymph node enlargement (metastases, lymphoma, tuberculosis, histoplasmosis, sarcoidosis, pneumoconiosis)

Aortic aneurysm

Dilated venous structures (azygos, hemiazygos, superior vena cava)

Bronchogenic carcinoma

Bronchogenic cyst

Pericardial cyst

Mediastinal hemorrhage/inflammation/lipomatosis

Approach to Diagnostic Imaging

■ 1. Plain chest radiograph

- Detects and determines precise compartment of a mediastinal mass but does little to characterize it (with the exception of peripheral calcification in an aneurysm or bronchogenic cyst)

■ 2. Computed tomography

- Definitive imaging study for determining the origin and extent of a mass and its underlying characteristics
- With contrast enhancement, highly accurate in differentiating among fatty, cystic, and soft-tissue masses and aneurysms

■ 3. Magnetic resonance imaging

- Equivalent to CT in confirming the presence and location of a mediastinal mass
- Less effective than CT for assessing tracheal involvement by a mass or for demonstrating calcification
- Superior to CT for distinguishing tumor from fibrosis and in patients in whom the use of iodinated contrast material is contraindicated

 Caveat: False-positive results may occur because of the relatively low spatial resolution of MRI, which may result in an inability to distinguish between a group of normal-sized nodes and a single enlarged node.

Mediastinal Mass (Posterior)

Presenting Signs and Symptoms

Asymptomatic and incidental finding on plain chest radiograph

Common Causes

Neurogenic tumor
Vertebral lesion (trauma, infection, tumor)
Esophageal lesion (dilatation, neoplasm, diverticulum, duplication cyst)
Hiatal hernia
Lymphoma
Aortic aneurysm (descending portion)
Bochdalek hernia

Approach to Diagnostic Imaging

■ 1. Plain chest radiograph

- Detects and determines precise compartment of a mediastinal mass but otherwise does little to characterize the mass (can show bone erosion in neurogenic tumor or air in a hiatal or Bochdalek hernia)

■ 2. Barium swallow

- Indicated if there is clinical suspicion of an esophageal lesion or hiatal hernia

■ 3. Computed tomography

- Definitive imaging study for defining the origin and extent of the mass and for determining its underlying characteristics
- With contrast enhancement, highly accurate in differentiating among fatty, cystic, and soft-tissue masses and aneurysms

■ 4. Magnetic resonance imaging

- Equivalent to CT in confirming the presence and location of a mediastinal mass
- Less effective than CT for showing calcification
- Superior to CT for showing the spinal cord and in patients in whom the use of iodinated contrast material is contraindicated

Metastases (Pulmonary)

Presenting Signs and Symptoms

Most are asymptomatic and only detected incidentally during staging or follow-up of patients with a known malignancy

Develop in up to one-third of patients with cancer

Only demonstrable metastatic site in about one-half of patients with metastatic spread of tumor

May produce shortness of breath in those with lymphangitic spread

Common Primary Sites of Tumor

Breast
Lung
Kidney
Thyroid
Head and neck
Melanoma

Approach to Diagnostic Imaging

■ 1. Plain chest radiograph

- Preferred screening technique (detects most metastases greater than 15 mm in diameter)
- May fail to detect smaller nodules (because of overlying ribs or blood vessels) and nodules in specific areas (lung apices, inferior recesses just above dome of diaphragm, subpleural region)
- Linear lower lobe interstitial disease is a sign of lymphangitic carcinomatosis

■ 2. Computed tomography

- Often detects small (3–10 mm), otherwise occult metastases (especially those located peripherally and in the subpleural region)
- Smooth and/or nodular thickening of interlobular septa and bronchovascular structures is seen in lymphangitic carcinomatosis
- Unfortunately, high sensitivity of CT leads to potential problem of false-positive examinations (granulomas, intrapulmonary lymph nodes, or even pulmonary vessels on end are sometimes erroneously interpreted as metastases)
- Best imaging modality for following the response of metastases to chemotherapy

Note: Although resolution of nodules indicates a positive response, persistent nodular opacities representing sterilized tumor deposits may be seen after successful treatment of metastatic seminoma, choriocarcinoma, or hypernephroma.

▪ 3. PET/CT

- ▪ Superior to CT alone is detecting metastases in non-enlarged lymph nodes and distinguishing reactive nodes from those with metastatic involvement
- ▪ Also allows distinction between granulomas and lung metastases when lesions >10 mm diameter
- ▪ Helps guide tissue sampling of abnormal lymph nodes or lung nodules to confirm the presence of metastatic disease

▪ 4. Radionuclide thyroid scan (total body)

- ▪ Highly specific and more sensitive than plain chest radiographs for detecting thyroid carcinoma metastatic to the lung

Indications for CT If Plain Chest Radiograph Is Normal

- ▪ 1. High propensity of tumor spread to lung (melanoma, testicular carcinoma, choriocarcinoma, head and neck tumors)

   Caveat: Common primary tumors of the lung, breast, colon, prostate, and cervix have a low propensity of spread to the lungs.

- ▪ 2. Presence of metastases would alter treatment (usually by cancellation of planned extensive surgery)
  - ▪ Radical amputation for osteosarcoma
  - ▪ Extensive lymph node dissection for melanoma
  - ▪ Lobectomy or radiofrequency ablation for presumed solitary metastasis or several (<5) nodules

■ 3. Effective therapy available for metastases (osteogenic sarcoma, choriocarcinoma, nonseminomatous testicular tumors, renal cell carcinoma, certain functioning thyroid carcinomas)

 Caveat: The detection of pulmonary metastases is of no clinical significance if there is no effective treatment for metastases or if there already are obvious extrathoracic metastases.

Pleural Effusion

Presenting Signs and Symptoms

Pleuritic pain

Dyspnea

Often asymptomatic and discovered as incidental finding on chest radiograph

Decreased or absent breath sounds, percussion dullness, and decreased motion of hemithorax

Common Causes

Congestive heart failure (usually bilateral but larger on the right)

Neoplasm (primary or metastatic lung cancer, lymphoma)

Pneumonia/abscess

Ascites

Pancreatitis (usually left-sided)

Tuberculosis

Pulmonary embolism (small)

Mixed connective tissue disease (lupus, rheumatoid arthritis)

Trauma (hemothorax)

Approach to Diagnostic Imaging

▪ 1. Plain chest radiograph

- Preferred initial imaging technique that can show classic blunting or meniscus appearance at the lateral and posterior costophrenic angles, apical cap, or increased opacity of the hemithorax without obscuring of vascular markings
- Large effusions may opacify an entire hemithorax and shift the mediastinum to the opposite side
- Subpulmonic effusions may be detected by an unusually lateral position of the top of the diaphragmatic contour on upright films, or an abnormal density interposed between the gastric fundus and the apparent left hemidiaphragm
- Lateral decubitus projection (affected side down), can determine whether pleural fluid is free or loculated and estimates the amount of the effusion

▪ 2. Computed tomography

- Procedure of choice for determining the status of the underlying lung parenchyma in a patient with extensive pleural effusion (e.g., may detect lung abscess, pneumonia, or bronchogenic carcinoma that is obscured on plain radiograph)
- Limited value in differentiating transudates from chylous effusions; exudates may show pleural enhancement on contrast studies (a specific but not sensitive finding)

■ 3. Ultrasound

- Readily available for bedside imaging in severely ill patients in whom a lateral decubitus projection cannot be obtained
- Best technique for identifying and localizing a loculated effusion as an echo-free or hypoechoic fluid collection separate from the lung and chest wall that may mimic a mass on plain radiographs
- May permit demonstration of an exudate as a complex, septated pattern or a homogeneously echogenic appearance
- Permits marking of the chest wall for thoracentesis (may be performed under ultrasound guidance in difficult cases)

Pneumoconioses

Presenting Signs and Symptoms

Insidious onset of decreased pulmonary function (related to occupational exposure to inorganic dusts)

Common Types

Silicosis
Asbestosis
Coal worker's pneumoconiosis
Talcosis

Approach to Diagnostic Imaging

■ 1. Plain chest radiograph

- Preferred initial imaging technique that may demonstrate a broad spectrum of chronic changes in the lung parenchyma and pleura

---

Note: There may be poor correlation between the extent of radiographic findings and the degree of alteration in pulmonary function.

■ 2. Computed tomography

- More sensitive than plain chest radiography for detecting subtle changes, but not usually necessary for clinical evaluation

Pneumomediastinum

Presenting Signs and Symptoms

Most often asymptomatic
Chest pain

Common Causes

Spontaneous
Trauma (injury to chest wall, bronchus, trachea, lung)
Iatrogenic (surgery or instrumentation of the esophagus, trachea, bronchi, or neck; overinflation during anesthesia and respiratory therapy)
Extension of gas from the neck or abdomen
Asthma (primarily in children)
Rupture of the esophagus (e.g., Boerhaave's syndrome)
Hyaline membrane disease (extension of pulmonary interstitial emphysema)

Approach to Diagnostic Imaging

■ 1. Plain chest radiograph

- Preferred imaging technique for detecting gas separating the medial margin of the pleura from the mediastinal contents or interposed between the heart and diaphragm
- Can show any associated pneumoperitoneum or gas within the soft tissues of the neck

> **Note:** The clinical concern in patients with pneumomediastinum includes development of a pneumothorax, which can have dire consequences in patients whose respiratory status is already compromised, and the possibility of esophageal or tracheobronchial disruption that requires urgent surgical repair.

■ 2. Computed tomography

- Can be helpful in identifying the source of pneumomediastinum in patients with suspected esophageal or tracheobronchial disruption

Pneumonia

Presenting Signs and Symptoms

Cough with sputum production
Fever and chills
Chest pain and dyspnea

Predisposing Factors

Viral respiratory infection
Cigarette smoking
Chronic obstructive pulmonary disease
Alcoholism
Loss of consciousness
Dysphagia with aspiration
Hospitalization or institutionalization
Surgery/trauma
Heart failure
Immunosuppressive disorders and therapy
Central obstructing neoplasm (e.g., bronchogenic carcinoma)

Approach to Diagnostic Imaging

■ 1. Plain chest radiograph

- ■ Preferred initial imaging technique to show the various patterns of opacification within the lung
- ■ Best imaging modality for identifying potential complications (empyema, extensive atelectasis, and focal or diffuse dissemination of the primary infection)

- If the retrocardiac area cannot be assessed on a portable image, a repeat chest radiograph should be obtained using abdominal technique to detect any increased opacification behind the heart or silhouetting of the left hemidiaphragm

---

Notes: The mere presence of an opacity in a patient with fever or chest pain does not necessarily indicate the presence of an infectious process. Atelectasis, neoplasm, pulmonary embolism or infarction, and atypical pulmonary edema can all mimic pneumonia both clinically and radiographically.

Pneumonia may exist in the presence of a normal radiograph (especially with atypical organisms and those pneumonias that develop in immunocompromised hosts).

Frequent radiographs after acute pneumonia should not be obtained in the normal population (unnecessary cost and radiation exposure), unless there is some clinical reason to warrant serial studies. Symptoms usually resolve, even though the radiographic opacity may be unchanged and persistent. However, in an *immunocompromised* patient in whom clinical manifestations may be depressed, serial chest radiographs are justified, as they may be the only means of following the results of a course of therapy.

■ 2. Computed tomography
- May be indicated if there is incomplete clearing of an opacity or clinical suspicion of either postobstructive pneumonia distal to an endobronchial lesion or a secondary lung abscess
- In patients with extensive chronic pulmonary disease, the presence of ground-glass opacification may indicate an acute inflammatory process that cannot be detected on plain chest radiographs

Pneumonia in AIDS Patients

Presenting Signs and Symptoms

Cough with sputum production
Fever and chills
Chest pain and dyspnea

Predominant Organisms

Pneumocystis jiroveci (formerly *Pneumocystis carinii*)
Histoplasma
Cytomegalovirus
Cryptococcus
Aspergillus
Toxoplasma
Varicella

Approach to Diagnostic Imaging

■ 1. Plain chest radiograph

- Preferred imaging technique to show the various patterns of opacifications within the lung
- Best imaging modality for identifying potential complications (empyema, extensive atelectasis, focal or diffuse dissemination of the primary infection)

Notes: The mere presence of an opacity in a patient with fever or chest pain does not necessarily indicate the presence of an infectious process. Atelectasis, neoplasm, pulmonary embolism or infarction, and atypical pulmonary edema can all mimic pneumonia both clinically and radiographically.

The radiograph may be normal, even though there is clinical evidence of pneumonia. Conversely, in immunocompromised patients, there may be extensive radiographic findings with minimal clinical manifestations. Therefore, in this population, serial chest radiographs are justified because they may be the only means of following a course of therapy (as opposed to the normal population, in which frequent radiographs after acute pneumonia should not be obtained).

■ 2. High-resolution computed tomography

- Can detect subtle interstitial or nodular opacities in patients with normal plain radiographs (e.g., Pneumocystis pneumonia, invasive aspergillus infection)
- Helps direct site and mode of sampling for stains/culture

Pneumothorax

Presenting Signs and Symptoms

Range from asymptomatic to sudden, sharp chest pain, severe dyspnea, shock, and life-threatening respiratory failure

Pain may be referred to corresponding shoulder, across the chest, or over the abdomen (simulating acute coronary occlusion or acute abdomen)

Markedly depressed or absent breath sounds

Shift of mediastinum to opposite side and ipsilateral diaphragmatic depression (with large or tension pneumothorax)

Common Causes

Spontaneous (rupture of small, usually apical bleb)

Trauma (penetrating or blunt, rib fracture, tracheobronchial injury)

Complication of mechanical ventilation (barotrauma)

Chronic obstructive pulmonary disease

Chronic pulmonary disease (e.g., sarcoidosis, Langerhan's cell histiocytosis)

Pneumocystis jiroveci pneumonia (formerly *Pneumocystis carinii*)

Lung abscess with bronchopleural fistula

Rupture of the esophagus (Boerhaave's syndrome)

Iatrogenic (surgery, lung or pleural biopsy, thoracentesis, central line placement)

Approach to Diagnostic Imaging

■ 1. Plain chest radiograph

- Preferred initial imaging technique that shows apical and lateral air without peripheral lung markings and separated from normal lung by a sharp pleural margin
- May show underlying bullous or interstitial changes consistent with chronic obstructive pulmonary disease or any chronic interstitial lung disorder

Notes: Pneumothorax is best seen on an expiration film.

In patients on mechanical ventilation for ARDS, a small pneumothorax on a supine film may present subtly as a loculated collection in a subpulmonic or paracardiac location. In such cases, abnormal lucency over the upper abdomen or an unusually deep and lucent costophrenic sulcus may be the only findings on supine radiography.

 Caveat: The visceral pleural line of a pneumothorax may be mimicked by skin folds (resulting from compression of redundant skin by the radiographic cassette). A true visceral pleural line is recognized by (a) the identification of a line, not the edge of a skin fold; (b) a pneumothorax usually extends over the lung apex, whereas a skin fold rarely does so, and (c) vascular markings are usually visible peripheral to a skin fold and should not be seen in a pneumothorax. The visceral pleural line may also be mimicked by bullae (it is necessary to detect the thin curvilinear walls that are concave rather than convex or parallel to the chest wall).

■ 2. Computed tomography

- More sensitive than plain chest radiographs for detecting a pneumothorax, but rarely necessary. Nevertheless, anterior pneumothorax is not uncommonly detected on CT scans of trauma and critically ill patients undergoing CT scans for other indications.
- May be required to differentiate pneumothorax from bullous disease and in patients in whom an anterior pneumothorax is suspected on a supine radiograph but who cannot undergo upright or lateral decubitus films
- In a patient undergoing CT for abdominal trauma, routine sections through the chest may be obtained to detect a subtle pneumothorax that might not be evident on conventional supine radiographs

Pulmonary Edema: Cardiac versus Noncardiac (Permeability)

Types of Edema

■ 1. Cardiac

- Low-protein transudate due to increased hydrostatic pressure generated across the capillary membrane that initially accumulates in the connective tissues surrounding the blood vessels and secondary pulmonary lobules

■ 2. Noncardiac

- Protein-rich exudate that accumulates in the extravascular space as a consequence of increased microvascular permeability. Because of inherent disruption of the alveolocapillary membrane in this condition, water may not flow into the loose connective tissue but may directly flood the alveolar space.

Note: Clearance of the protein-rich exudate is slower than that of the nonproteinaceous transudate.

Approach to Diagnostic Imaging

■ 1. Plain chest radiograph

- Can distinguish between cardiac and noncardiac (permeability) edema in about 80% of patients using the following criteria:

	Cardiac	*Noncardiac*
Major Signs		
Kerley lines	Present	Unusual
Pleural effusions	Present	Unusual
Cardiomegaly	Present	Unusual
Opacities in lung	Diffuse	Patchy and peripheral
Minor Signs		
Air bronchograms	Rare	Often present
Hilar haze	Present	Infrequent
Peribronchial cuffs	Present	Unusual

Pulmonary Fibrosis

Presenting Signs and Symptoms

Often asymptomatic except for insidious onset of exertional dyspnea

Cough (if secondary bronchial infection)

Anorexia, weight loss, fatigue, weakness, vague chest pains

Cyanosis, cor pulmonale, clubbing (severe disease)

Common Causes

Idiopathic (idiopathic pulmonary fibrosis)

Collagen vascular diseases (scleroderma, rheumatoid arthritis)

Sarcoidosis

Langerhan's cell histiocytosis

Occupational exposure (asbestosis)

Hypersensitivity pneumonitis (chronic)

Immunosuppressive and antineoplastic drugs (busulfan, bleomycin, methotrexate, cyclophosphamide)

Approach to Diagnostic Imaging

■ 1. Plain chest radiograph

- Preferred initial imaging technique to show characteristic pattern of prominent reticular opacities, rounded opacities, and small cystic lesions (honeycombing), as well as evidence of secondary pulmonary hypertension and cor pulmonale

 Caveat: Chest films may be normal even in the presence of significant symptoms or functional abnormalities.

■ 2. High-resolution computed tomography

- ■ More sensitive than plain chest radiographs for detecting pulmonary fibrosis and suggesting the correct histologic diagnosis

---

Note: Lung biopsy may be needed if the imaging findings and clinical course do not indicate the precise diagnosis.

Pulmonary Embolism

Presenting Signs and Symptoms

Nonspecific tachypnea, dyspnea, and hemoptysis; pleuritic chest pain in pulmonary embolism with infarction

Major Risk Factors

Prolonged bed rest

Hypercoagulable state (protein C or S, antithrombin III deficiency, lupus anticoagulant)

Recent surgical procedure

Recent myocardial infarction or chronic congestive heart failure

Deep venous thrombosis in the veins of the pelvis or proximal lower extremities

Indwelling venous catheter

Approach to Diagnostic Imaging

■ 1. Plain chest radiograph

- Usually normal (may be nonspecific opacity, pleural effusion, atelectasis, or elevation of the hemidiaphragm indistinguishable from other pulmonary or pleural processes)
- Classic pleural-based, wedge-shaped opacity (Hampton's hump) is seen in a minority of cases with pulmonary infarction
- Uncommon findings of focal oligemia (Westermark's sign) and enlargement of the ipsilateral pulmonary artery (Fleischner's sign)
- Essential for accurate interpretation of radionuclide ventilation–perfusion lung scan

■ 2. Contrast-enhanced computed tomography

- Has replaced V/Q lung scanning in most institutions as the preferred imaging modality for detecting and excluding pulmonary emboli
- Shows a pulmonary embolus as a filling defect within the pulmonary artery or as an abrupt cutoff (complete obstruction) of a pulmonary artery branch

Note: Multi-detector CT reduces the effect of respiratory and motion artifact on scan quality and improves detection of subsegmental emboli.

■ 3. Radionuclide ventilation–perfusion (V/Q) lung scan

- Previously the most frequently performed noninvasive imaging study for detecting clinically significant pulmonary emboli
- If the perfusion study is *normal,* significant embolization is excluded and no further studies are needed
- If segmental or larger perfusion defects are present with normal ventilation in these areas (V/Q mismatch), there is a high likelihood of pulmonary embolism

 Caveat: There may be a relatively large number of indeterminate examinations, especially in patients with chronic obstructive pulmonary disease or parenchymal abnormalities seen on plain chest radiographs.

■ 4. Pulmonary arteriography

- Most definitive study ("gold standard") that shows pulmonary emboli as intraarterial filling defects or abrupt cutoff (complete obstruction) of pulmonary vessels
- Rarely used today. Only indicated if non-invasive tests are inconclusive and the patient is either a surgical candidate (for venous occlusion or embolectomy) or at extremely high risk for anticoagulation

---

Note: Doppler ultrasound, magnetic resonance venography, or delayed indirect CT venography of the lower extremities may be employed as noninvasive procedures to search for supporting evidence of venous clots if the diagnosis of pulmonary embolus is equivocal.

Pulmonary Nodule (Solitary)

Presenting Signs and Symptoms

Asymptomatic

Incidental finding on a chest radiograph

Detected on chest computed tomography performed for screening or for another indication

Common Causes

Benign nonneoplastic process (granuloma, arteriovenous malformation)

Benign neoplastic process (hamartoma)

Primary bronchogenic carcinoma

Solitary metastasis (colon, breast carcinoma)

Peripheral carcinoid tumor (rare)

Age Effect on Malignancy in Solitary Nodule

Younger than age 30: Cancer risk is less than 1%

Ages 30–45: Cancer risk is about 15%

Older than age 50: Cancer risk is 50%

Radiographic Criteria for Benignity

Central dense, laminated, or popcorn calcification

Feeding artery and draining vein indicating an arteriovenous malformation

No growth demonstrated on serial chest films over 2 years (comparison studies must be aggressively sought and reviewed)

Characteristic features of rounded atelectasis (volume loss, feeding bronchovascular structures, association with pleural thickening, enhancement on contrast CT similar to atelectatic lung)

Approach to Diagnostic Imaging

■ 1. Computed tomography

- May show central dense, laminar, or popcorn calcification indicating benignancy that was not evident on plain chest radiograph, or fat within a nodule that is highly specific for hamartoma
- May show additional nodules not visible on plain chest radiograph (suggesting metastases)
- Detects any hilar or mediastinal metastases
- Permits percutaneous fine-needle aspiration biopsy of peripheral lesions as an alternative to thoracotomy for establishing a definite diagnosis

Note: The use of multidetector CT scanners with improved spatial resolution has led to the increased detection of small (< 1 cm) nodules. For solid nodules less than 4 mm in diameter, no further evaluation is necessary unless the patient has a significant smoking history or other risk factor for primary or metastatic cancer. In this case, follow-up CT examination is recommended at 12 months. If the nodule is unchanged, no further follow-up is needed. For solid nodules 4–10 mm in diameter, various regimens of follow-up are recommended depending on the size of the nodule and the cancer risk of the patient.

■ 2. PET/CT scanning

- Pulmonary malignancies >10mm in diameter almost invariably demonstrate higher FDG radio-isotope uptake than normal lung parenchyma and benign nodules, due to their increased metabolic activity. Therefore, a negative PET study has a high negative predictive value in excluding malignancy (exceptions include bronchoalveolar cell and well-differentiated adenocarcinomas, peripheral carcinoid tumors). However, because inflammatory nodules and hamartomas can demonstrate increased metabolic activity on PET, biopsy should be performed for the majority of PET-positive nodules to determine whether they are malignant.

■ 3. Percutaneous fine-needle aspiration biopsy

- Cost-effective alternative to thoracotomy for establishing a definite diagnosis of a peripheral lesion (25% pneumothorax rate, although chest tube required in ≤5%; false-negative rate of about 5–10% in patients with carcinoma)

Sarcoidosis

Presenting Signs and Symptoms

Asymptomatic (hilar and mediastinal lymphadenopathy discovered incidentally on a routine chest radiograph)

Constitutional symptoms (fever, weight loss, anorexia, fatigue)

Erythema nodosum and other skin lesions

Uveitis

Hypercalcemia/hypercalciuria

Variety of symptoms involving the cardiac, respiratory, musculoskeletal, and central nervous systems

Common Causes

Unknown

Approach to Diagnostic Imaging

■ 1. Plain chest radiograph

- Preferred initial imaging technique that may demonstrate characteristic bilateral hilar and right paratracheal lymphadenopathy and a diffuse reticular pulmonary infiltration that may accompany or follow the lymphadenopathy

■ 2. High-resolution computed tomography

- More sensitive than plain chest radiographs for detecting parenchymal pulmonary changes and enlarged lymph nodes in regions that are invisible on plain radiographs
- Classic appearance is nodular thickening of bronchovascular and subpleural interstitium, often associated with hilar and mediastinal lymphadenopathy

Note: Although good correlation has been shown between the CT findings and pulmonary function, clinically this imaging modality is not as important as the response to therapy and pulmonary function tests.

Trauma (Blunt Chest)

Approach to Diagnostic Imaging

■ 1. Plain chest radiograph

- Preferred initial imaging study that can confirm suspected clinical diagnoses (tension pneumothorax, hemothorax, pulmonary contusion)
- Can diagnose or suggest other injuries that may be difficult to detect by clinical examination (mediastinal and pericardial hemorrhage, diaphragmatic rupture, and bronchial, esophageal, or pulmonary parenchymal laceration)
- May be obtained rapidly during acute resuscitation efforts

■ 2. Computed tomography

- Far more sensitive than plain chest radiograph for detecting chest wall injuries, pneumothorax, ruptured diaphragm or esophagus, aortic or great vessel injury, pleural or pericardial hemorrhage, and pulmonary contusion and laceration

Note: A pneumothorax detected by CT that is not seen on plain radiographs is generally benign, except when the patient is to receive positive pressure ventilation.

- Effective in demonstrating mediastinal hemorrhage and for the direct assessment of aortic injury in a patient whose plain chest radiographs are equivocal or of suboptimal quality

---

Note: A contrast-enhanced CT scan of the mediastinum that is of good quality and unequivocally normal indicates that the aorta is intact and thus precludes the need for aortography.

■ 3. Aortography

- Although highly accurate for the diagnosis of aortic injury, this modality is time consuming, not as rapidly available as CT, and is rarely necessary when multi-detector CT is normal.

Tuberculosis

Presenting Signs and Symptoms

Varies from asymptomatic exposure to fever, productive cough, and night sweats

Approach to Diagnostic Imaging

■ 1. Plain chest radiograph

- Preferred imaging technique to show the various patterns of opacification within the lungs
- Lordotic projection can be obtained if the apical region is not clearly seen on the frontal view.
- Although fibrotic changes are consistent with old tuberculous disease, it is necessary to demonstrate the absence of change from images obtained at least 2 years previously to unequivocally exclude activity of the process.

Wegener's Granulomatosis

Presenting Signs and Symptoms

Paranasal sinus congestion and pain

Nasal mucosal ulcerations (with consequent secondary bacterial infection)

Serous or purulent otitis media with hearing loss

Cough, hemoptysis, dyspnea, pleuritis

Glomerulonephritis (renal failure is major cause of death)

Common Causes

Unknown

Approach to Diagnostic Imaging

■ 1. Plain chest radiograph

- Preferred initial imaging technique to demonstrate the characteristic multiple and bilateral thick-walled cavitating lung lesions (50% of patients), as well as a pattern of diffuse or nodular opacities that may simulate metastases

■ 2. Computed tomography

- Best imaging technique for detecting mucosal and submucosal lesions in the tracheobronchial tree (seen almost exclusively in women) that produce irregular narrowing of the airway lumen
- Demonstrates cavitary nodules or masses and diffuse alveolar opacification patterns of lung involvement

3

BREAST

D. David Dershaw

Palpable Breast Mass

Approach to Diagnostic Imaging

■ 1. Mammography

- Procedure of choice for determining whether a palpable mass is unequivocally benign (e.g., calcified fibroadenoma, intramammary lymph node, oil cyst, lipoma) or probably malignant, thus avoiding any unnecessary workup. In young women (under age 30) the initial assessment of a palpable breast mass should be done with ultrasound; if a cyst is detected, no imaging with radiation exposure is needed.

- If the palpable mass is suspicious for malignancy, the primary purpose of mammography is to assess the affected breast for the extent of disease and the contralateral breast for clinically occult but mammographically suspicious abnormalities that should be biopsied concurrently. Mammography is also needed to assist in determining whether needle biopsy should be done using stereotaxis or sonography for guidance. Additionally, if stereotaxis is indicated, mammography it is useful to decide on the approach to the lesion.

Note: The palpable mass is generally indicated by placing a radiopaque marker over the site to ensure that the palpable abnormality is included on available images, and to determine whether it corresponds to any mammographic lesion that is visualized.

■ 2. Ultrasound

- Indicated as a confirming procedure if physical examination or mammography suggests that the palpable mass may represent a simple cyst or intramammary lymph node. Can be diagnostic of a simple (benign) cyst or intramammary lymph node if rigid interpretive criteria are used. When biopsy is indicated, ultrasound is needed to determine whether needle biopsy can be done under sonographic, rather than mammographic (i.e., stereotactic) guidance.

- Can be used instead of needle aspiration to determine if a palpable mass, which cannot be characterized by mammography, is a simple cyst.

 Caveat: US *cannot* provide a definitive diagnosis of other solid or complex masses.

■ 3. Fine-needle aspiration biopsy

- Provides material for definitive cytologic examination. Limited by a high insufficient sampling rate and best done with a cytologist present to determine the adequacy of the sample. Inadequate samples and suspicious cytologic results require repeat biopsy.

■ 4. Core biopsy

- Provides material for definitive histologic examination. Repeat biopsy done surgically is required if the diagnosis is ductal atypia. Many also believe this should be done with lobular carcinoma in situ, lobular atypia, and radial scar. Ductal carcinoma in situ found at core biopsy may have an invasive component at surgery.

Note: Although usually done for nonpalpable lesions, image-guided needle biopsy may be performed when a lesion is palpable. This is most common when biopsy guided by palpation has failed to make a diagnosis, when a lesion is only vaguely palpable, or when an imaging lesion is present and it is uncertain whether this corresponds to the palpable mass.

Nipple Discharge

Causes

BENIGN (90%)

Normal (physiological)
Papilloma (intraductal)
Mammary duct ectasia
Fibrocystic changes

MALIGNANT (10%)

Approach to Diagnostic Imaging

Note: Nipple discharge that requires workup is unilateral, serous or serosanguinous, and spontaneous. Although rarely diagnostic, imaging workup of nipple discharge enables definitive localization of the site of the symptomatic intraductal lesion so that biopsy can be performed.

■ 1. Galactography (ductography)

- Primary modality to evaluate the source and cause of nipple discharge. After cannulation of the duct from which fluid has been expressed and the injection of contrast material, mammography is performed to image the duct.
- Although ductography often can localize the site of the lesion causing a nipple discharge, the procedure does not determine whether the ductal lesion is benign or malignant. Careful evaluation of the opacified duct is necessary, because multiple lesions may be present.

- The failure rate of the procedure may be high. It cannot be done if there is no discharge, and duct cannulation may be difficult to perform if there is nipple distortion, prior surgery, or absence of any major duct ectasia associated with the discharge.

■ 2. Ultrasound

- Directed sonography may be helpful in imaging the lesion if palpation of a single point in the breast expresses a nipple discharge

Note: If imaging identifies a lesion, image-guided biopsy or preoperative localization can be done.

Screening

Routine Mammography

American Cancer Society Guidelines

For women age 40 and older, *yearly* mammograms are recommended

---

Note: In several screening studies involving asymptomatic women, about 40% of cancers were detected by mammography but not physical examination. Conversely, about 10% of cancers were evident only on physical examination. Therefore, physical examination and mammography should be considered as *complementary* procedures.

 Caveat: US and MRI are *not* used as screening procedures for breast cancer in the general population, but these modalities are valuable in diagnosing the disease. Thermography, diaphanography, transillumination, or other techniques should *never* be used for the screening or diagnosis of breast disease.

Screening Outcomes

Note: The following outcomes are representative for 1,000 asymptomatic women undergoing bilateral screening mammography for the first time.

70–100 (7–10%) will be recalled for more studies (magnification or other special views; US)

15–20 (1.5–2%) will require biopsy, with carcinoma detected in only 20–45% of recommended biopsies

5–7 (0.5–0.7%) will have cancer detected (1–3/1,000 women screened)

Recall rate, biopsy rate, and cancer detection rate will be approximately 50% of subsequent screening examinations

Note: Of cancers detected on screening studies, more than 40% will be minimal (ductal carcinoma in situ of any size, invasive cancer <1 cm), and more than 75% will be node-negative.

High-Risk Screening

Women at significantly increased risk for breast cancer may undergo more aggressive screening than that recommended for the general population. This includes annual mammography before age 40, and/or additional annual screening with MRI (or US if MRI is not available). Women in this group include those with:

Family history of breast cancer in premenopausal women (especially first-degree relatives and bilateral cancers)

Genetic risk for breast cancer

BRCA-positive women

Cowden's syndrome

Other rare disorders

Biopsy diagnosis of atypia or lobular carcinoma in situ

Personal history of breast cancer

Mantle radiation for Hodgkin's disease

BI-RADS Categories in Breast Imaging Reports

The Breast Imaging Reporting and Data System (BIRADS) of the American College of Radiology is a quality assurance tool designed to standardize mammographic reporting, reduce confusion in breast imaging interpretations, and facilitate outcome monitoring.

Inclusion of the BI-RADS category in the mammogram report is required under federal law in the United States. BI-RADS categories are also commonly included in reports of US and MRI studies of the breast.

Assessment Categories and Recommended Follow-up

0   Incomplete study; additional imaging evaluation needed
1   Negative; routine annual mammogram recommended
2   Benign finding; routine annual mammogram recommended
3   Probably benign; short-term follow-up (usually six-months) recommended (lesion has less than 2% chance of malignancy)
4   Suspicious; biopsy recommended (lesion has 2–75% chance of malignancy, usually in 20–50% range)
5   Probably malignant; biopsy recommended (lesion has >75% chance of being malignant)
6   Known carcinoma; mammogram shows cancer that has been previously diagnosed

Breast Cancer

Presenting Signs and Symptoms

Asymptomatic (detected by screening)

Variable clinical manifestations, including mass, breast enlargement, nipple discharge, nondescript thickening, lymphedema (peau d'orange), skin or nipple retraction, and evidence of matted or fixed axillary or supraclavicular lymph nodes

Although pain is the most common breast complaint by women, it is rarely a presenting symptom of breast cancer

Risk Factors

MAJOR

See High-Risk Screening (page 115)

MINOR

(Same screening regimen as for general population.)

Long, uninterrupted menstrual history (especially early in life)

Early menarche

Late menopause

No pregnancy carried to term or no pregnancy at a young age

Note: Other less-significant factors that may increase a woman's risk include obesity, alcohol consumption, middle class and upper middle class life style (including college education), and lack of physical exercise.

Approach to Diagnostic Imaging

■ 1. Mammography

- Procedure of choice for detecting nonpalpable cancer because it demonstrates microcalcifications and can show small malignant masses. Although highly sensitive (demonstrates up to 90% of breast cancers) it has low specificity. Because mammography frequently underestimates the extent of cancer within a breast, preoperative staging for conservation may require additional imaging studies.
- Facilitates preoperative needle/wire localization of nonpalpable lesions for which surgery is being performed
- Screening tool to detect synchronous, unsuspected cancer in the contralateral breast
- Provides definitive diagnosis for selected benign lesions, including calcified fibroadenoma, intramammary lymph node, oil cyst and some other forms of fat necrosis, and lipoma

■ 2. Ultrasound

- If mammography suggests a cyst, indicated to make the critical distinction between a simple cyst (always benign and requiring no further workup) and a complex or solid mass (may be malignant and requiring further investigation)
- Sufficiently characterizes an intramammary lymph node to establish the diagnosis

 Caveat: US *cannot* provide a definitive diagnosis of other solid or complex masses.

- May be used to preoperatively stage extent of disease within the breast if MRI is not available
- Helpful to characterize palpable lesions that are not seen mammographically and to determine if blood flow is present in a lesion using Doppler (absence of flow supports a benign diagnosis)

■ 3. Magnetic resonance imaging

- Generally considered the best tool for staging the extent of tumor in the breast. May be indicated before breast conservation surgery, especially for women with invasive lobular carcinoma, large areas of ductal carcinoma in situ, or dense breasts that are not well assessed by mammography
- For women undergoing breast conservation in whom the initial attempt at therapeutic surgery showed positive margins, it is appropriate to obtain an MRI to assess the extent of residual disease in the breast before repeat surgery is performed
- For women with probably metastatic breast cancer in axillary nodes but no evidence of primary tumor on physical examination or mammography, MRI should be used to attempt to detect a tumor within the breast
- Women undergoing MRI for known breast cancer should also have the contralateral breast imaged, because otherwise-unsuspected cancer is detected in 9%
- Occasionally, MRI is useful to further assess an indeterminate mammogram, sonogram, or physical examination

■ 4. Fine-needle aspiration biopsy

- Provides material for definitive cytologic examination. Cannot differentiate invasive from in situ carcinoma. Some surgeons will not do conservation or mastectomy based on fine-needle aspiration and require core or surgical biopsy.
- Can be performed by palpation or using imaging guidance (stereotactic, US, MRI)

■ 5. Core biopsy

- Provides material for definitive histologic examination
- Can be performed with stereotactic, US, or MRI guidance

Recurrent Breast Cancer after Mastectomy

Common Causes

Although this can be due to residual foci of glandular tissue or malignancy, recurrence at the mastectomy site is considered metastatic disease (stage IV cancer)

Approach to Diagnostic Imaging

 Caveat: Literature and clinical course generally do not support screening of the reconstructed breast, because early diagnosis of disease at this site does not improve the rate of cure. Disease at this site is considered metastatic. Any palpated lump is generally biopsied, and superficial recurrence typically can be easily palpated.

■ **1. Mammography**

- If a mass in the reconstructed breast is suspected to represent fat necrosis, mammography may identify typical changes that allow a definitive diagnosis. Otherwise, the findings are nonspecific.

■ **2. Ultrasound**

- Can characterize margins, internal structure, and vascularity of the mass, as well as chest wall involvement
- Useful for biopsy guidance

■ 3. Magnetic resonance imaging

- Can characterize margins, vascularity and internal structure of a mass, as well as chest-wall involvement

■ 4. Computed tomography

- May aid in evaluating the extent of recurrent disease and visualizing tissue posterior to an implant, as well as assessing the axilla, chest wall, and lungs for metastatic disease

■ 5. Core biopsy

- Provides material for definitive histologic examination

Note: Routine mammographic screening of the *contralateral* breast is essential.

Breast Implant Assessment for Rupture

Presenting Signs and Symptoms

Pain, lump(s), abrupt or gradual contour change, or volume decrease

Often asymptomatic (especially intracapsular ruptures)

Approach to Diagnostic Imaging

■ 1. Mammography

- Detects all cases of saline implant rupture by demonstrating collapse of the implant shell (saline is resorbed)
- Detects many cases of extracapsular silicone implant rupture by demonstrating free silicone in the breast or axilla
- Cannot detect intracapsular silicone implant rupture
- Detects malignancy, either clinically occult or associated with a palpable lump

Note: In addition to routine mammographic views, the study of a breast with an implant requires additional implant displacement views. The presence of an implant, especially when superficial to the pectoralis muscle, compromises mammographic screening.

■ 2. Magnetic resonance imaging

- Preferred technique because of its ability to image silicone separately from breast tissue. The presence of multiple implants or a multi-chambered implant can simulate intracapsular rupture.
- MRI for a suspected implant complication is technically different from a study to evaluate breast parenchyma. No intravenous contrast is given. The ordering physician should specify that an examination for implant assessment is being requested.
- More sensitive and specific than breast US or mammography for detecting a ruptured implant. May be used to confirm the results of other studies before surgery if the mammographic or breast US findings do not support the clinical impression.

■ 3. Ultrasound

- May be used if MRI not available, although it is more operator-dependent and may not visualize posterior to the implant
- High false positive rate, so that MRI confirmation of rupture may be required before surgery. Most valuable for evaluating a palpable lump in a woman with an implant to determine whether it is due to rupture or a parenchymal lesion.

4

CARDIOVASCULAR

U. Joseph Schoepf

Vascular

Angina Pectoris

Presenting Signs and Symptoms

Episodes of precordial discomfort or pressure, typically precipitated by exertion and relieved by rest or sublingual nitroglycerin

Common Cause

Atherosclerotic coronary artery disease

Risk Factors

Elevated serum cholesterol
High cholesterol intake
Tobacco smoking (primarily cigarettes)
Diabetes mellitus
Hypertension
Strong family history

Approach to Diagnostic Imaging

■ 1. Radionuclide myocardial perfusion scan

- SPECT scanning has a specificity and sensitivity approaching 95% for detecting areas of myocardial ischemia as perfusion defects on stress testing that fill in during an examination performed with the patient at rest

Note: Perfusion defects that are stable during both stress and rest examinations usually represent areas of infarction.

■ 2. Coronary arteriography

- Indicated when angioplasty or bypass surgery is being considered
- Evaluates the extent and severity of disease (percentage of stenosis involving one, two, or three vessels)
- Left ventricular angiogram can be obtained to evaluate wall motion (if not contraindicated by potential adverse effects of additional volume of contrast material on renal or ventricular function)

Note: Wall motion can also be assessed by radionuclide techniques or echocardiography.

■ 3. Coronary CT angiography

- Can be considered in patients with atypical chest pain or equivocal findings on other tests (e.g., stress test, radionuclide myocardial perfusion scan)
- High negative predictive value, so that a normal or near-normal coronary CT angiogram reliably rules out significant coronary artery stenosis. There are some limitations with this technique for grading the degree of stenosis in affected vessels.

- Parameters of cardiac function, both global (ejection fraction, end diastolic volume, end systolic volume, stroke volume myocardial mass) and regional (segmental wall motion), can be evaluated using functional cine-loop analysis of retrospectively ECG-gated coronary CT angiography scans

■ 4. Radionuclide gated blood pool studies

- To evaluate the ejection fraction because of the important relationship between ventricular function and prognosis

■ 5. Angioplasty

- Interventional technique in which inflation of a balloon-tipped catheter at the site of a stenotic atherosclerotic lesion can rupture the intima and media and dramatically dilate the obstruction
- Coronary artery stents can be deployed to keep stenotic vessels patent

---

Note: This is an alternative to bypass grafting in patients with suitable anatomic lesions (risk is comparable to surgery).

Evaluating Postsurgical Patency of Bypass Grafts

■ 1. Coronary CT angiography

- Useful in patients undergoing repeat bypass surgery for pre-surgical evaluation of graft location and operative planning

Claudication

Presenting Signs and Symptoms

Deficient blood supply to muscles during exercise (initially intermittent, may proceed to continuous pain at rest)

Common Cause

Atherosclerotic vascular disease

Approach to Diagnostic Imaging

■ 1. Ultrasound with color Doppler

- Preferred noninvasive imaging technique to demonstrate the presence of atherosclerotic plaques and assess the degree of luminal stenosis

■ 2. Ankle-brachial index (ABI)

- A blood pressure cuff is inflated at the ankle, and a systolic measurement (A) is taken by Doppler at the posterior tibial and dorsalis pedis arteries. An arm pressure (B) is also recorded, and the ratio (ABI) is computed:

Normal	1.0
Claudication	0.5–1.0
Rest pain/ulceration	<0.5

Note: Diabetics usually have an artificially elevated ABI due to calcified tibial vessels.

■ 3. Arteriography

- Indicated if surgery or angioplasty is contemplated to more precisely define the location and extent of a lesion and assess the status of the peripheral runoff vessels

■ 4. MR or CT angiography

- Using contrast enhancement, these rapidly evolving and continually improving techniques provide excellent non-invasive imaging of the entire lower extremity run-off and are considered the methods of choice for diagnostic purposes (i.e., if no immediate intervention is planned). MRA and CTA have similar accuracy for diagnosing lesions and for follow-up after interventional or surgical procedures. The choice of MRA versus CTA should be based on local expertise and patient-specific contraindications (e.g., pacemaker, renal insufficiency).

■ 5. Interventional radiology (percutaneous transluminal angioplasty)

- PTA, with or without stenting, is generally considered the treatment of choice for focal iliac lesions
- Nearly as durable as aorto-bifemoral bypass grafting with much lower morbidity
- Excellent technical success with PTA below the pelvis, but not as durable as surgical bypass procedures

Congestive Heart Failure

Common Causes

Left ventricular failure (e.g., secondary to ischemic heart disease)

Valvular heart disease (stenosis or regurgitation)

Pulmonary venoocclusive disease

Congenital heart disease

Approach to Diagnostic Imaging

■ 1. Plain chest radiograph

- Demonstrates the classic findings of indistinct vascular markings, progressive redistribution of venous blood flow to the lungs (cephalization), and Kerley B lines (edematous thickening of the interlobular septa at the periphery of the lungs)

■ 2. Echocardiography, magnetic resonance imaging, or cardiac computed tomography

- Can evaluate the dimensions of the left ventricle and other cardiac chambers, ejection fraction, and wall-motion dysfunction

- Echocardiography and MRI can be used to assess the presence and severity of incompetence or stenosis of heart valves

- Echocardiography, CT, and MRI can accurately detect the presence of pericardial effusion, intracardiac thrombi, and cardiac tumors
- CT and MRI can accurately diagnose congenital anomalies
- Cardiac CT can assess for coronary artery disease if an ischemic etiology is suspected

 Caveat: Care must be taken to avoid volume overload induced by iodinated contrast in patients with severe congestive heart failure.

Peripheral Ischemia (Acute)

Presenting Signs and Symptoms

Sudden onset of severe pain, coldness, numbness, and pallor of a portion of an extremity

Absent pulses distal to the obstruction

Common Causes

Embolization (from the heart, a proximal atherosclerotic plaque, or an aneurysm)

Acute thrombosis on preexisting atherosclerotic disease

Approach to Diagnostic Imaging

■ 1. Arteriography

- Demonstrates the precise site of obstruction and permits therapeutic thrombolysis of the clot

 Caveat: Lytic therapy is contraindicated in patients with active bleeding; recent gastrointestinal bleeding, central nervous system surgery, or stroke; intracranial tumor; or nonviable extremity. Complications include bleeding, puncture site hematoma, pericatheter thrombus formation, and distal embolization.

■ 2. MR or CT angiography

- Using contrast enhancement, MRA and CTA provide excellent non-invasive imaging of the entire lower extremity run-off. In acute ischemia, they can demonstrate the precise site and nature of obstruction and aid in selecting the appropriate therapeutic approach (e.g., endovascular versus surgical embolectomy, thrombolysis, primary bypass)

 Caveat: In acute cases of limb-threatening ischemia, cross-sectional imaging must be used only in experienced centers and when readily available in order to avoid delays in treatment.

Cardiac Tumors

Presenting Signs and Symptoms

Protean findings of fever, elevated erythrocyte sedimentation rate, anemia, weight loss, syncope, and embolic symptoms

Left atrial lesions may mimic rheumatic valvular disease

Common Causes

Metastases (breast, lung, lymphoma, melanoma)

Myxoma

Rhabdomyoma, lipoma, fibroma

Sarcoma

Approach to Diagnostic Imaging

■ 1. Echocardiography (especially transesophageal)

- In left atrial myxoma, confirms the presence of a mass that often prolapses into the left ventricle during diastole

■ 2. Magnetic resonance imaging

- Excellent for detecting direct extension of a lesion, intracardiac metastases, and pericardial involvement in suspected malignant cardiac tumor

■ 3. Computed tomography

- Demonstrates invasion of the heart by noncardiac tumors of the lung or mediastinum
- Cardiac CT is diagnostic of most intracardiac masses (including blood clots)

Cardiomyopathy (Restrictive)

Presenting Signs and Symptoms

Congestive heart failure
Arrhythmias
Heart block

Common Causes

Infiltrative disorders (amyloid, glycogen storage disease, mucopolysaccharidoses, hemochromatosis, sarcoidosis, tumor infiltration of the myocardium)
Endomyocardial fibrosis (highly prevalent in the tropics)

Approach to Diagnostic Imaging

■ 1. Plain chest radiograph

- Typically shows a normal-sized (or even small) heart with pulmonary venous congestion

■ 2. Echocardiography, magnetic resonance imaging, or cardiac computed tomography

- Shows normal systolic and diastolic function, myocardial hypertrophy, and often dilatation of the atria
- Demonstrates a normal pericardium, thus permitting differentiation from constrictive pericarditis (in which the pericardium is thickened)
- CT is highly accurate in differentiating restrictive cardiomyopathy from constrictive pericarditis (pericardial thickening/ calcifications)
- MRI can demonstrate abnormal texture or tissue infiltration of the myocardium (e.g., in patients with amyloidosis or sarcoidosis)

Cardiomyopathy (Congestive)

Presenting Signs and Symptoms

Congestive heart failure (may be right-sided or left-sided dominance or biventricular involvement)

Common Causes

Chronic diffuse myocardial ischemia (coronary artery disease)

Infection (especially coxsackievirus, Chagas disease)

Toxins or drugs (ethanol, doxorubicin, cocaine, psychotherapeutic drugs)

Granulomatous disease (sarcoidosis, giant cell myocarditis, Wegener's granulomatosis)

Metabolic disease (endocrinopathies, lipid or glycogen storage diseases, uremia)

Nutritional deficiencies (beriberi, selenium deficiency, kwashiorkor)

Connective tissue disorders

Approach to Diagnostic Imaging

■ 1. Plain chest radiograph

- Demonstrates global cardiomegaly and evidence of congestive failure

> **Note:** Detection of coronary artery calcification may be a clue to an underlying ischemic cause.

■ 2. Echocardiography

- Shows dilated, hypokinetic cardiac chambers with reduced fractional shortening, while excluding primary valvular disease or segmental wall-motion abnormalities (seen in discrete myocardial infarcts)

■ 3. Magnetic resonance imaging or cardiac computed tomography

- Demonstrate dilatation of specific cardiac chambers and abnormal cardiac function. MRI can show abnormal texture or tissue infiltration (e.g., storage diseases) of myocardial tissue. Contrast-enhanced cardiac MRI can detect foci of myocarditis

 Caveat: Care must be taken to avoid volume overload induced by iodinated contrast in patients with severe congestive heart failure.

■ 4. Radionuclide scan

- Gated myocardial scintigraphy demonstrates abnormal ejection fractions and times; gallium scanning can detect acute myocarditis

Cardiomyopathy (Hypertrophic)

Presenting Signs and Symptoms

Chest pain
Syncope
Palpitations
Exertional dyspnea
Congestive heart failure

Note: Sudden death occurs in about 50% of patients (overall mortality rate about 2–3% per year).

Common Causes

Longstanding hypertension
Familial (autosomal dominance with variable penetration)
Obstructive (subaortic or midventricular)

Approach to Diagnostic Imaging

■ 1. Plain chest radiograph

- Deceptively normal-looking in about 50% of patients (because hypertrophy occurs at the expense of the ventricular cavities)
- May demonstrate left atrial enlargement (commonly due to mitral regurgitation)
- May show right ventricular enlargement or an unusual shape of the cardiac silhouette that is not diagnostic of any specific disorder (e.g., neither a valvular lesion nor pericardial effusion)

■ 2. Echocardiography

- Preferred noninvasive modality that permits measurement of the thickened ventricular walls and allows differentiation among the different subgroups
- Often permits quantitation of the degree of obstruction of the outflow tract (an important determinant of the effectiveness of treatment)

■ 3. Cardiac computed tomography or magnetic resonance imaging

- Alternative modalities to echocardiography
- Permit diagnosis and quantitation of the severity of hypertrophic cardiomyopathy (allows assessment of all areas of the myocardium and is not subject to the imaging limitations of echocardiography)
- Can provide information on particular patterns and functional consequences of myocardial hypertrophy (e.g., in patients with hypertrophic obstructive cardiomyopathy)
- May evaluate left ventricular mass and provide indices of left ventricular function, as well as exclude other cardiac and noncardiac abnormalities

Congenital Heart Disease

Presenting Signs and Symptoms

Broad spectrum of murmurs, shunts, alterations in systemic and pulmonary blood flow, and altered workloads of specific cardiac chambers

Cyanosis (in right-to-left shunts)

Risk Factors

Chromosomal defects (trisomy 13, 18, 21; Turner's syndrome; Holt-Oram syndrome)

Maternal illness (diabetes mellitus, systemic lupus erythematosus)

Environmental exposure (e.g., thalidomide)

History of congenital heart disease in a first-degree relative

Common Types

Atrial septal defect

Ventricular septal defect

Patent ductus arteriosus

Total anomalous venous return

Persistent truncus arteriosus

Transposition

Endocardial cushion defect

Tetralogy of Fallot

Hypoplastic right heart syndrome

Coarctation of the aorta

Approach to Diagnostic Imaging

BEFORE BIRTH

■ 1. Prenatal ultrasound

- May permit the diagnosis of some serious defects during pregnancy (thus offering the parents the option of discontinuing the pregnancy or permitting the physician and parents to make realistic plans for the labor, delivery, and care of the child)

■ 2. Fetal MRI

- May permit the diagnosis of some serious defects during pregnancy and may aid in decision making and planning of intrauterine corrective surgery

AFTER BIRTH

■ 1. Plain chest radiograph

- Initial imaging study for assessing the pulmonary vasculature, size of the main pulmonary artery, size and position of the aorta (especially whether it is right-sided), and size and contour of the cardiac silhouette

■ 2. Echocardiography

- Plays a prominent role in the initial imaging evaluation of congenital heart disease

■ 3. Magnetic resonance imaging

- MRI and MRA have become the primary modality for imaging most congenital heart disease because of the ability to show directly both morphologic and functional anomalies in multiple planes

■ 4. Computed tomography

- Computed tomography is increasingly used for diagnosing congenital cardiovascular disorders
- With modern CT technology, patient sedation or general anesthesia are generally no longer necessary. The risk of radiation exposure in pediatric patients must be weighed against the risks of sedation or anesthesia, which are often required for pediatric cardiovascular MRI

■ 5. Angiocardiography

- Definitive (but invasive) study

Note: Some authors recommend angiocardiography only if surgery is contemplated.

Cor Pulmonale

Presenting Signs and Symptoms

Exertional dyspnea
Angina pectoris
Syncope

Common Causes

Chronic obstructive pulmonary disease
Pulmonary fibrosis
Acute or chronic pulmonary embolism
Primary pulmonary hypertension
Pulmonary venoocclusive disease
Extrapulmonary diseases affecting pulmonary mechanics
(morbid obesity, chest wall deformities, neuromuscular
disease)

Approach to Diagnostic Imaging

■ 1. Plain chest radiograph

■ Usually shows a normal-sized heart or only mild
cardiomegaly, but there may be enlargement of
the right ventricle and right atrium

Note: Plain films may be relatively insensitive indi-
cators of right ventricular enlargement because
hyperinflation of the lungs and bullae may distort
the position of the heart in these patients.

- Characteristic prominence of the main and central pulmonary arteries with rapid tapering (pruning) so that the lung periphery appears oligemic

---

Note: The lungs usually will show evidence of chronic obstructive pulmonary disease or interstitial fibrosis (i.e., right ventricular failure secondary to pulmonary arterial or parenchymal disease).

■ 2. Echocardiography

- Indicated to evaluate the degree of function of the left ventricle (as well as the degree of enlargement of the right atrium and right ventricle)

■ 3. Computed tomography

- Can be useful for diagnosing the etiology of cor pulmonale (e.g., chronic obstructive pulmonary disease, pulmonary fibrosis, acute or chronic pulmonary embolism)
- Shows the degree of enlargement of the right atrium and right ventricle for assessment of right cardiac strain
- Can be used for patient selection and surgical planning prior to thromboendarterectomy

Myocardial Infarction

Presenting Signs and Symptoms

Deep substernal chest pain (described as an aching or pressure) that often radiates to the back, jaw, or left arm

Pain similar to that of angina pectoris but usually more severe, long lasting, and relieved only a little or briefly by rest or nitroglycerin

Symptoms of left ventricular failure, pulmonary edema, shock, or significant arrhythmia may dominate the clinical appearance

About 20% of acute myocardial infarctions are silent (or not recognized as an illness by the patient)

Elevation of myocardial enzymes in the serum

Common Causes

Atherosclerotic coronary artery disease

Coronary artery dissection as a complication of aortic dissection (type A)

Approach to Diagnostic Imaging

■ 1. Plain chest radiograph

- Useful as a baseline for assessing pulmonary venous congestion

Direct Infarct Imaging

 Caveat: The diagnosis of myocardial infarction is usually evident from the patient's history and confirmed by electrocardiogram and enzyme studies. In such cases, immediate catheter arteriography with subsequent percutaneous angioplasty (with or without stenting) and/or thrombolysis is indicated for myocardial reperfusion. Infarct imaging is indicated if the clinical, laboratory, and electrocardiographic findings are equivocal; if there has been recent cardiac surgery or trauma; or prior to revascularization therapy to assess myocardial viability.

■ 1. Radionuclide imaging

- Can demonstrate areas of myocardial infarction and usually determine whether they are acute or remote
- Radionuclide viability imaging can differentiate viable from non-viable myocardium and predict the success of revascularization therapy
- Enables assessment of global and regional myocardial function for evaluating the functional consequences of ischemia and patient prognosis

■ 2. Magnetic resonance imaging

- Can directly demonstrate areas of myocardial infarction and differentiate between subendocardial and transmural extension
- MR viability imaging can differentiate viable from non-viable myocardium and predict the success of revascularization therapy
- Enables assessment of global and regional myocardial function for evaluating functional consequences of ischemia and patient prognosis

■ 3. Coronary CT angiography

- Can be considered in patients with acute chest pain, equivocal findings at electrocardiography, and negative enzyme studies
- High negative predictive value of a normal or near-normal coronary CT angiography study, which reliably rules out coronary artery disease as a reason for acute chest pain
- CT can diagnose other thoracic disease (e.g., aortic dissection, pulmonary embolism, pneumonia) as an alternative cause for acute chest pain

Note: Echocardiography is often performed to assess the function of the right and left ventricles, as well as to detect the 10–20% incidence of cardiac-wall clots that alter clinical management.

Endocarditis (Infective)

Presenting Signs and Symptoms

Insidious onset of low-grade fever, night sweats, fatigue, malaise, weight loss

New regurgitant murmur and signs of valvular insufficiency

Chills and arthralgia

Emboli may produce stroke, myocardial infarction, flank pain and hematuria, abdominal pain, or acute arterial insufficiency in an extremity

Petechial hemorrhages and Osler's nodes

Predisposing Factors

Rheumatic heart disease

Congenital heart disease (ventricular septal defect, tetralogy of Fallot)

Prosthetic heart valve

Intravenous drug abuse

Central venous line

Approach to Diagnostic Imaging

■ 1. Echocardiography

- Procedure of choice (particularly with transesophageal echocardiography) for demonstrating the characteristic vegetations on affected heart valves

> **Note:** Transesophageal echocardiography should be repeated after 6 weeks of intravenous antibiotic therapy for infective endocarditis.

■ 2. Cardiac computed tomography or magnetic resonance imaging

- Can assess vegetations and complications of valvular disease and valve surgery (e.g., perivalvular aneurysm)
- CT accurately demonstrates valve calcifications.
- Complementary to echocardiography, especially in seriously ill patients who cannot lie flat (i.e., the table can be tilted)

Valvular Heart Disease

Presenting Signs and Symptoms

Murmur and clinical symptoms vary, depending on the precise valve involved and whether there is predominant stenosis or regurgitation

Common Causes

Rheumatic fever
Congenital heart disease
Infectious endocarditis

Approach to Diagnostic Imaging

■ 1. Plain chest radiograph

- Inexpensive imaging technique to show enlargement of the entire heart or specific chambers, valvular calcification, and any evidence of pulmonary vascular congestion

■ 2. Echocardiography

- More precisely demonstrates any chamber enlargement or wall thickening and the precise size of the orifices of affected valves
- Doppler flow studies can assess the degree of regurgitation
- Transesophageal ultrasound (TEE) is the method of choice for diagnosing infectious vegetations in patients with a high clinical suspicion

■ 3. Computed tomography or magnetic resonance imaging

- Cine MRI demonstrates and quantitates the regurgitation of blood across an incompetent valve
- Cardiac CT and MRI can be used to assess for vegetations and complications of valvular disease and valve surgery (e.g., perivalvular aneurysm)
- CT accurately demonstrates valve calcifications

Cardiac Tamponade

Presenting Signs and Symptoms

Cardiogenic shock (low cardiac output and low systemic arterial pressure)

Tachycardia

Dyspnea and orthopnea

Usually elevated systemic venous pressure (prominent neck veins) and pulmonary venous pressure

Distant heart sounds

Pericardial rub

Pulsus paradoxus (accentuation of the normal inspiratory decline in systemic systolic blood pressure greater than 10 mm Hg)

Mechanism

Pericardial effusion or hemorrhage under tension causing compression of the cardiac chambers and compromising diastolic filling

Approach to Diagnostic Imaging

■ 1. Plain chest radiograph

- Demonstrates rapid enlargement of the cardiac silhouette with relatively normal-appearing vasculature

■ 2. Echocardiography

- Modality of choice not only to demonstrate the accumulation of a large amount of pericardial fluid but also to show septal shift, paradoxic septal motion, diastolic collapse of the right ventricle, and cyclic collapse of the atria

■ 3. Computed tomography or magnetic resonance imaging

- Cardiac CT and MRI can detect pericardial fluid, while density measurements and signal characteristics can characterize pericardial fluid as serous or hemorrhagic/proteinaceous
- Can often diagnoses the precise etiology of acute pericardial tamponade (e.g., type A aortic dissection)

Constrictive Pericarditis

Presenting Signs and Symptoms

Elevation of ventricular diastolic, atrial, pulmonary, and systemic venous pressures (unlike tamponade, the ventricular venous pressure, or ejection fraction, is usually preserved)

Dyspnea and orthopnea (prolonged elevation of pulmonary venous pressure)

Hypervolemia, engorgement of neck veins, pleural effusion, hepatomegaly, ascites, peripheral edema (elevated systemic venous pressure)

Kussmaul's sign (inspiratory swelling of neck veins), which is absent in tamponade

Common Causes

Postpericardiotomy (although the pericardium is usually partly resected after coronary artery bypass grafting)

Viral infection (especially coxsackievirus B)

Tuberculosis

Uremia

Radiation

Neoplastic involvement

Rheumatoid arthritis

Idiopathic

Approach to Diagnostic Imaging

■ 1. Plain chest radiograph

- Demonstrates characteristic pericardial calcification in 50% of patients (as well as pleural effusions, small atria, a flat or straightened right heart border, and dilated superior and inferior vena cava and azygos vein)

■ 2. Magnetic resonance imaging or cardiac computed tomography

- Preferred imaging techniques to show the abnormally thick pericardium (which permits the distinction of constrictive pericarditis from restrictive cardiomyopathy)
- MRI can show that the pericardial thickening represents fibrosis; CT can detect pericardial calcifications

---

Note: Although echocardiography can show the thickened pericardial wall, the findings are not as specific as in the case of pericardial fluid.

Pericardial Effusion

Presenting Signs and Symptoms

Severity of symptoms varies greatly depending on the
underlying cause, the rate at which the pericardial
fluid accumulates, and the total amount present

Milder symptoms include chest pain and a friction rub;
large effusions may lead to congestive heart failure and
shock

Faint, distant heart sounds on auscultation

Common Causes

Idiopathic

Infection

Autoimmune (systemic lupus erythematosus, rheumatoid
arthritis, scleroderma)

Dressler's and postpericardiotomy syndromes

Neoplasm (lymphoma, lung or breast metastases)

Drug-induced (procainamide, hydralazine, phenytoin)

Uremia

Myxedema

Congestive heart failure

Trauma

Approach to Diagnostic Imaging

■ 1. Plain chest radiograph

- Suggests the diagnosis if there is a rapid increase in the size of the cardiac silhouette on serial chest films (especially when the lungs remain clear)

> **Note:** A rapid increase in heart size related to congestive heart failure is generally associated with pulmonary venous congestion.

■ 2. Echocardiography

- Procedure of choice for demonstrating as little as 50 mL of pericardial fluid (normal, 20 mL) as a posterior sonolucent collection

■ 3. Computed tomography or magnetic resonance imaging

- Cardiac CT and MRI can detect loculated pericardial effusions that can be difficult to diagnose with echocardiography. CT density measurements and signal characteristics at MR can characterize pericardial fluid as serous versus hemorrhagic/proteinaceous.

Aneurysm (Thoracic Aorta)

Presenting Signs and Symptoms

Asymptomatic
Symptoms related to secondary compression
  Stridor, wheezing (trachea and bronchi)
  Dysphagia (esophagus)
  Venous obstruction of the upper extremities, head, and neck (superior vena cava)
  Hoarseness (recurrent laryngeal nerve)
Substernal or back pain

Common Causes

Atherosclerosis
Syphilis
Mycosis
Connective tissue disorders (Marfan's and Ehlers-Danlos syndromes)

Approach to Diagnostic Imaging

■ 1. Plain chest radiograph

- Demonstrates contour abnormalities and tortuosity of the thoracic aorta, as well as calcification within its wall

 Caveat: It may be difficult to distinguish a thoracic aneurysm from other mediastinal masses.

■ 2. Computed tomography or magnetic resonance imaging

- Preferred methods for initial evaluation and follow-up
- Accurately demonstrates vessel diameter, mural thrombus, calcifications, degree of luminal patency, mass effects on adjacent mediastinal structures, and evidence of leakage or rupture
- CT is superior to MRI for showing calcifications within the wall of an aneurysm
- Three-dimensional image post-processing based on CT or MRI can be used to demonstrate the relationship of an aneurysm to the arch vessels and for surgical planning

■ 3. Aortography

- Indicated only for preoperative planning when it is vital to know the relationship between the aneurysm and the great vessels and coronary arteries, as well as the vascular supply to the spinal cord

---

Note: Aortography is unreliable for assessing the size of an aneurysm, as it only visualizes the patent portion of the lumen and cannot show the extent of mural thrombus.

Aneurysm (Abdominal Aorta)

Presenting Signs and Symptoms

Most are asymptomatic and discovered incidentally on routine physical examination or plain abdominal radiograph

Pulsatile mass

Severe abdominal pain and hypotension (if rupture)

Common Causes

Atherosclerosis

Trauma

Arteritis syndromes

Connective tissue disorders (Marfan's syndrome, cystic medial necrosis)

Syphilis

Approach to Diagnostic Imaging

 Caveat: Any patient with a pulsatile abdominal mass and hypotension should proceed directly to surgery without any intervening imaging study.

■ 1. Ultrasound

- Most cost-effective initial imaging technique to show dilatation of the aorta to greater than 3 cm and the presence of intraluminal clot
- Serial examinations can be easily performed to follow aneurysm size in patients who are not considered surgical candidates at the time

 Caveat: Ultrasound has limited ability to consistently show the proximal and distal extent of an aneurysm and its relationship to the surrounding retroperitoneal structures (required prior to elective surgical repair).

■ 2. CT angiography

- Modality of choice for initial diagnosis, monitoring of aneurysm size, surgical planning, and assessment of therapeutic success (e.g., detection of endoleaks after endovascular repair)
- More accurate than ultrasound for determining the true diameter of an aneurysm, its longitudinal extent, and relationship to branch vessels (renal and iliac arteries) prior to surgical or endovascular repair, particularly if three-dimensional image post-processing is performed

■ 3. Magnetic resonance imaging

- Alternative to CTA
- Especially useful in patients with depressed renal function (because MR contrast is not nephrotoxic)

■ 4. Aortography

- Traditionally, the preoperative procedure of choice for determining the number of renal arteries and their relationship to the aneurysm, as well as the patency of the visceral, renal, external iliac, and femoral arteries (factors that may modify the surgical approach and define additional procedures required to decrease postoperative morbidity)
- Because aortography outlines only the aortic lumen, it underestimates the true size of an aneurysm if its wall is lined with thrombus.

Note: The ability of newer, less invasive techniques such as CT and MRA to demonstrate the extent of an aneurysm and the patency of other vessels has substantially reduced the need for preoperative aortography, which now is rarely required for this purpose.

 Caveat: There is *no* indication for plain lateral radiographs of the abdomen to detect calcification in the wall of an aneurysm (very low sensitivity).

Aneurysm (Peripheral)

Presenting Signs and Symptoms

Limb ischemia (due to thrombus within the aneurysm)
Signs of distal embolization
Gangrene

Common Causes

Atherosclerosis
Trauma
Mycosis
Complication of vascular surgery

Approach to Diagnostic Imaging

■ 1. Ultrasound with color Doppler

- Preferred initial imaging procedure to detect a peripheral aneurysm (most commonly involving the popliteal artery) and assess its size

---

Note: CT or MR angiography may be employed to evaluate a suspected aneurysm.

■ 2. CT or MR angiography

- Modalities of choice for evaluating the location and size of aneurysms and their relationship to surrounding anatomy prior to surgical therapy. Both can assess thrombus formation; CTA can detect calcification.

■ 3. Arteriography

- Ordinarily performed as part of endovascular therapy
- Covered stents inserted via the femoral artery may be used instead of bypass grafting to repair aneurysms

Aortic Dissection

Presenting Signs and Symptoms

Sudden, severe, tearing substernal chest pain with radiation to the back

Frequent migration of pain from the original site as the dissection extends along the aorta

Aortic insufficiency murmur

Absent or asymmetric major arterial pulses

Neurologic complications (stroke, paraparesis, or paraplegia from spinal cord ischemia; ischemic peripheral neuropathy from abrupt occlusion of an artery supplying a limb)

Predisposing Factors

Hypertension

Connective tissue disorders (Marfan's and Ehlers-Danlos syndromes)

Bicuspid aortic valve

Coarctation of the aorta

Trauma

Granulomatous arteritis

Pregnancy (cause of 50% of dissections in women younger than age 40)

Previous aortic surgery or arterial catheterization

Approach to Diagnostic Imaging

■ **1. Plain chest radiograph**

- Demonstrates mediastinal widening in up to 90% of patients and frequently a left pleural effusion
- Localized bulging of the aortic contour indicates the likely site of origin of a dissection

■ **2. Computed tomography**

- Preferred initial imaging study in acutely ill patients
- Shows the classic double-barrel aorta (opacification of both the true and false lumens) and intimal flap (linear filling defect within the aortic lumen)
- Can precisely evaluate the origin and extent of the dissection, as well as the degree of involvement of major arterial trunks arising from the aorta (including the coronary arteries) and end-organs

■ **3. Magnetic resonance imaging**

- Equally accurate as CT, but often difficult to obtain in severely ill patients who require life-support systems and close monitoring
- Functional MRI can assess the severity of any aortic insufficiency

■ **4. Aortography**

- Infrequently used for diagnostic purposes (largely replaced by CTA and MRA). Performed as part of endovascular repair.

Peripheral Occlusive Vascular Disease

Presenting Signs and Symptoms

Intermittent claudication that progresses to pain at rest
Coolness and numbness of the affected extremity
Nonhealing ulcers
Gangrene
Diminished pulses distal to the area of narrowing

Vessels Primarily Involved

Superficial femoral artery
Aortoiliac system
Trifurcation vessels
Popliteal artery

Approach to Diagnostic Imaging

■ 1. Ultrasound with color Doppler

- Preferred noninvasive imaging technique to demonstrate the presence of atherosclerotic plaques and assesses the degree of luminal stenosis

■ 2. Ankle-brachial index (ABI)

- A blood pressure cuff is inflated at the ankle, and a systolic measurement (A) is taken by Doppler at the posterior tibial and dorsalis pedis arteries. An arm pressure (B) is also recorded, and the ratio (ABI) is computed.

Normal	1.0
Claudication	0.5–1.0
Rest pain/ulceration	<0.5

Note: Diabetics usually have an artificially elevated ABI due to calcified tibial vessels.

■ 3. Arteriography

- Indicated if surgery or angioplasty is contemplated
- More precisely defines the location and extent of a lesion and assesses the status of the peripheral runoff vessels

Note: MRA is rapidly improving and may eventually replace contrast arteriography for evaluating the peripheral vascular system.

■ 4. MR or CT angiography

- Using contrast enhancement, these rapidly evolving and continually improving techniques provide excellent non-invasive imaging of the entire lower extremity run-off and are considered the methods of choice for diagnostic purposes (i.e., if no immediate intervention is planned). They have similar accuracy for diagnosing lesions or post-interventional/post-surgical follow-up. The choice of MRA or CTA should be based on local expertise and patient contraindications (e.g. pacemaker, renal insufficiency).

■ 5. Interventional radiology (percutaneous transluminal angioplasty)

- Excellent alternative to surgery for dilating localized stenotic lesions (especially in the iliac arteries where the success rate approaches 95%)

Note: The success rate in arteries of the thigh and calf is about 50–60%.

Deep Venous Thrombosis

Presenting Signs and Symptoms

Asymptomatic (one-third of patients with symptomatic pulmonary emboli but no clinical signs of DVT will nevertheless have a lower extremity venous thrombus)

Variable combination of pain, edema, warmth, skin discoloration, and prominent superficial veins over the involved area

Delayed complications of dermatitis, ulceration, and varicosities

Common Causes

Stasis (postoperative, postpartum states; chronic illness)

Pregnancy or the use of oral contraception

Obesity

Hypercoagulability (malignant tumor, blood dyscrasia)

Endothelial injury (indwelling catheter, injection of irritating substance, septic phlebitis, thromboangiitis obliterans)

Prolonged immobilization with the legs dependent while traveling (especially on prolonged airplane flights)

Approach to Diagnostic Imaging

■ 1. Color Doppler ultrasound

- Preferred initial imaging modality (>95% accuracy) that can demonstrate lack of compressibility of the vein (indicating the presence of thrombus within it)

- Visualizes intraluminal thrombus itself and characteristic alterations in spontaneous flow that occur because of obstruction of the proximal veins

■ 2. Venography

- Traditional "gold standard" that can demonstrate the conclusive finding of a persistent filling defect within the lumen of a vein
- Other findings that are highly suggestive of DVT include abrupt termination of the contrast column within a vein, inability to opacify a major vein, and the formation of extensive collateral venous circulation

■ 3. Indirect CT venography

- Commonly performed in combination with CT pulmonary angiography for diagnosing pulmonary embolism
- Most useful for evaluating venous territories that are difficult to assess with Doppler ultrasound (e.g., pelvic veins)

Note: See Pulmonary Embolism (page 96).

Superior Vena Cava Syndrome

Presenting Signs and Symptoms

Progressive dilatation of the veins of the head and upper extremities

Edema and plethora of the face, neck, and upper torso

Cyanosis and conjunctival edema

Dizziness, syncope, headache

Respiratory distress (due to airway edema)

Note: If the obstruction occurs slowly, the formation of a compensatory collateral venous network may prevent the development of clinical symptoms.

Common Causes

Malignant neoplasm (primary bronchogenic carcinoma, lymphoma, metastases from breast carcinoma)

Mediastinal granulomatous or fibrosing disease

Long-term indwelling central venous catheter

Aortic aneurysm

Congenital anomalies

Approach to Diagnostic Imaging

- **1. Computed tomography or magnetic resonance imaging**
  - Preferred noninvasive methods to show both the proximal dilatation of the superior vena cava and its branches and the underlying cause of the obstruction

- **2. Venography**
  - Allows better definition of the superior vena cava and collateral vessels
  - Metallic stents are generally the preferred treatment for malignant obstruction of the SVC. These can be placed via a femoral vein puncture and usually provide relief of symptoms within several hours.

Thoracic Outlet Syndrome

Presenting Signs and Symptoms

Numbness, paresthesias, pain, and sensory and motor deficits in the hand, neck, shoulder, or arm (secondary to arterial, venous, or nerve compression)

Obliteration of the radial pulse on the involved side with 90° elevation and external rotation of the arm or with simultaneous hyperextension of the neck and turning of the head toward the affected side (if the artery is involved)

Intermittent cyanosis, edema, and thrombotic symptoms (if the vein is involved)

Common Causes

Congenital anatomic anomaly (cervical rib, abnormal insertion of the anterior scalene muscle on the first rib)

Aberrant healing of rib or clavicle fracture

Neoplasm

Approach to Diagnostic Imaging

■ 1. Plain chest radiograph

- Imaging study of choice to demonstrate a cervical rib or a tumor in the apex of the lung

■ 2. Arteriography or venography

- Studies performed in both the neutral position (arms at the sides) and in the position that reproduces the patient's symptoms may demonstrate kinking or partial obstruction of the subclavian artery or vein

■ 3. MR or CT angiography

- Studies performed in both the neutral position (arms at the sides) and in the position that reproduces the patient's symptoms may demonstrate kinking or partial obstruction of the subclavian artery or vein

5

GASTROINTESTINAL
Richard M. Gore

Ascites

Presenting Signs and Symptoms

Small amounts may be asymptomatic
Abdominal distension and discomfort
Anorexia, nausea, and early satiety
Respiratory distress (due to reduced lung volume)
Bulging flanks, fluid wave, shifting dullness
Spontaneous bacterial peritonitis

Common Causes

Cirrhosis
Neoplasm (hepatic cancer or peritoneal carcinomatosis)
Congestive heart failure
Tuberculosis (and other infections)
Hypoalbuminemia (nephrotic syndrome, protein-losing
enteropathy, malnutrition)

Approach to Diagnostic Imaging

■ 1. Ultrasound

- Mobile, echo-free fluid regions shaped by adjacent
  structures
- Smallest amounts (as little as 100 mL) in a supine
  patient appear first in the hepatorenal area
  (Morison's pouch), the superior right flank,
  and the cul-de-sac of the pelvis.

■ 2. Computed tomography

- More expensive, but may demonstrate the underlying abdominal disease process (if US fails to do so)
- May be able to distinguish ascites (water attenuation) from blood (higher attenuation) or chyle (lower attenuation)

 Caveat: Plain abdominal radiographs are *not* indicated because a large amount of fluid (800–1000 mL) must be present to be detected and the underlying cause is infrequently shown.

Constipation

Presenting Signs and Symptoms

Decrease in frequency of stools or difficulty in defecation

Common Causes

Acute

Bowel obstruction or adynamic ileus

Chronic

Neurologic dysfunction (diabetes, spinal cord disorder, parkinsonism, idiopathic megacolon)

Scleroderma

Drugs (anticholinergic agents, opiates, aluminum-based antacids)

Hypothyroidism

Cushing's syndrome

Hypercalcemia

Debilitating infection

Anorectal pain (fissures, hemorrhoids, abscess, proctitis)

Approach to Diagnostic Imaging

■ 1. Plain abdominal radiograph

- Detects mechanical bowel obstruction

■ 2. Computed tomography

- Better characterizes the site and cause of narrowing or obstruction of the bowel

■ 3. Radiopaque marker study

- A plain abdominal radiograph 5 days after the ingestion of radiopaque markers can indicate whether there is a significant delay in clearing the radiopaque material from the bowel

■ 4. CT colonography (virtual CT colonoscopy)

- ■ Excellent examination when performed by experienced radiologists familiar with the procedure, using up-to-date equipment and software that facilitates reading and avoids both false negative and false positive findings of polyps or cancer

■ 5. Defecography (evacuation proctography)

- ■ Dynamic study that can demonstrate mechanical abnormalities such as rectal intussusception, rectal prolapse, rectocele, or puborectalis sling dysfunction

Diarrhea

Presenting Signs and Symptoms

Increased volume, fluidity, or frequency of fecal discharges

Common Causes

Osmotic (lactase deficiency, polyvalent laxative abuse)

Secretory (viral or protozoal infection, bacterial toxins, castor oil, Zollinger–Ellison syndrome, prostaglandin therapy, vasoactive intestinal peptide)

Exudative (mucosal inflammation, necrosis, neoplasm)

Malabsorption (sprue, pancreatic insufficiency, bowel resection, Whipple's disease)

Altered intestinal motility (diabetes, hyperthyroidism, magnesium-containing laxatives, irritable bowel syndrome)

Approach to Diagnostic Imaging

■ 1. Computed tomography

- Excellent baseline study

> **Note:** Residual barium residual from a small bowel examination may remain in the bowel for a long time, particularly in elderly patients, precluding the performance of CT and prolonging hospital stay. Therefore, a baseline CT examination should be performed as the first, and often only required, imaging study.

■ 2. Small bowel study

- Relatively non-specific examination that requires frequent spot imaging and great expertise in interpretation

Dysphagia
(Difficulty Swallowing)

Presenting Signs and Symptoms

Difficulty initiating swallowing
Food sticking in the upper or middle esophageal region
Odynophagia (pain on swallowing)
Regurgitation
Aspiration

Common Causes

Carcinoma
Peptic or lye stricture
Achalasia
Scleroderma
Diffuse esophageal spasm
Cervical esophageal web
Lower esophageal (Schatzki's) ring
Neuromuscular disorder
Dysmotility (abnormal propulsion)

Approach to Diagnostic Imaging

■ 1. Barium swallow

- Imaged digitally or on video fast-sequence radiographs

 Caveat: Hyperosmolar water-soluble contrast should *not* be used because aspiration of this material causes increased fluid to enter the tracheobronchial tree and may lead to the development of pulmonary edema. If aspiration is a major concern, the examination can be performed with isotonic, iso-osmotic iodinated contrast material.

Gastrointestinal Bleeding (Chronic, Obscure Origin)

Presenting Signs and Symptoms

Anemia (iron deficiency)
Fecal occult blood/guaiac positive stools

Common Causes

Neoplasm (benign or malignant anywhere in the alimentary tube)
Peptic ulcer
Gastritis
Meckel's diverticulum
Angiodysplasia

Approach to Diagnostic Imaging

Note: In most cases, these patients initially undergo upper gastrointestinal endoscopy or optical colonoscopy rather than an imaging procedure.

■ **1. CT enterography or dedicated small bowel follow-through study**

- If *negative,* proceed to

■ 2. Capsule video-endoscopy

- The patient wears a belt with a data recorder for 8 h after swallowing a capsule containing a camera, transmitter, and four light-transmitting diodes. This technique can demonstrate small, superficial bleeding ulcers that cannot be detected by enteroclysis. Disadvantages include the cost, the difficulty in determining the location of an abnormality, the inability of the technique to be used in partial small bowel obstruction, and the long time required for the study to be read (more than 2 h) even by the most experienced gastroenterologist.

■ 3. Radionuclide scan for Meckel's diverticulum

- Isotope may collect in ectopic gastric mucosa

> **Note:** Endoscopy and colonoscopy can also be used to detect a source of chronic gastrointestinal bleeding, depending on the availability of physicians skilled in performing these techniques.

■ 4. CT angiography

- Arterial phase study can demonstrate the bleeding site if there is massive hemorrhage. However, in most cases it merely shows arteriovenous malformations, the most common cause of chronic bleeding in older patients.

Gastrointestinal Bleeding
(Acute Lower)

Presenting Sign and Symptom

Brisk rectal bleeding without blood in gastric aspirate

Common Causes

Diverticulosis
Angiodysplasia
Ischemic colitis
Hemorrhoids (diagnosed by proctoscopy)
Polyps/carcinoma (more frequently associated with chronic bleeding)

Approach to Diagnostic Imaging

■ 1. Radionuclide scan

- Most sensitive diagnostic study that can document active bleeding of as little as 0.05–0.1 mL/min as a focal area of increased radionuclide activity corresponding to extravasation of blood in the gastrointestinal tract
- Movement of the radionuclide proximally or distally indicates active bleeding. Lack of movement suggests an angiodysplasia, arteriovenous malformation, or vascular tumor

Note: If the radionuclide scan shows no evidence of an active bleeding site, there is *no* indication for arteriography.

■ 2. CT angiography

- If bleeding continues to be rapid (>0.5–1 mL/min), may show the precise bleeding site by demonstrating extravasation of contrast material into the lumen of the bowel or the tangled blood vessels of an angiodysplasia

■ 3. Arteriography

- Offers therapeutic options through transcatheter measures (embolization or vasoconstrictive agents) and may preclude the need for surgery (especially in diverticular hemorrhage)

> **Note:** Many patients have a positive radionuclide scan and a bleeding site demonstrated surgically but a *negative* arteriogram.

■ 4. Colonoscopy

- Indicated only if bleeding is minimal or has stopped, to search for underlying colonic pathology that *may* represent the bleeding site

> **Note:** Colonoscopy, although valuable for assessing chronic and subacute bleeding, is not the examination of choice for acute rapid bleeding because the presence of fresh blood and clots prevents an adequate view of the mucosa.

 Caveat: Unstable patients with massive hemorrhage should have emergency surgery without any diagnostic studies.

Gastrointestinal Bleeding (Acute Upper)

Presenting Signs and Symptoms

Hematemesis, melena, hematochezia
Blood in nasogastric aspirate

Common Causes

Peptic ulceration (duodenum, stomach, esophagus)
Gastric mucosal lesion (superficial erosions, stress ulcers)
Esophageal varices
Neoplasm
Mallory–Weiss tear

Approach to Diagnostic Imaging

■ 1. Endoscopy

- Procedure of choice that can permit precise visual identification of a lesion that is actively bleeding
- Offers therapeutic options (electrocautery or laser cautery, mechanical clips, tissue adhesives, or injection of sclerosing agents for varices)
- May be falsely negative if there is rapid bleeding, because large amounts of fresh blood and clots may obscure the underlying bleeding lesion

■ 2 Arteriography

- Indicated for patients with rapid bleeding (0.5–1 mL/min, but not if massive hemorrhage) in whom endoscopy is technically difficult
- Demonstrates extravasation of contrast material or an angiodysplasia
- Offers therapeutic options through transcatheter measures (embolization or infusion of vaso-constrictive agents); even if hemostasis fails or is only temporary, generally allows time for vascular volume replacement to stabilize the patient before surgery

■ 3. CT angiography

- Demonstrates vessels with great detail and may show site of bleeding, but lacks the therapeutic capability of catheter arteriography

---

Note: Introduction of barium into the gastrointestinal tract prevents the performance of endoscopy or computed tomography until the barium has cleared from the region of interest, which may take several days in elderly patients.

 Caveat: Patients with massive hemorrhage whose condition is unstable should have emergency surgery without any diagnostic studies.

Jaundice: Differentiation of Medical (Hepatocellular) from Surgical (Biliary Obstruction) Causes

Presenting Signs and Symptoms

Yellowing of skin and sclera
Abnormal liver enzymes
Dark urine and pale stools

Common Causes

Common duct stone
Pancreatic carcinoma
Cholangiocarcinoma
Primary hepatocellular dysfunction (alcoholism, hepatitis)

Approach to Diagnostic Imaging

■ 1. Ultrasound

- Preferred initial imaging technique for demonstrating dilated bile ducts (indicating biliary obstruction)
- May be equivocal or incomplete in obese patients or those with large amounts of intestinal gas

■ 2. Computed tomography

- Highly accurate for showing dilated bile ducts, as well as disease in adjacent structures (liver, porta hepatis, pancreas, adrenals, retroperitoneum)
- Not adversely affected by obesity or large amounts of intestinal gas

■ 3. Magnetic resonance cholangiopancreatography (MRCP)

- Preferred diagnostic approach if ERCP is likely to be unsuccessful, as in patients with surgical bypass procedures (Billroth II anastomosis, hepatojejunostomy) or those with acute pancreatitis (increased risk of complications from ERCP)

■ 4. Endoscopic retrograde cholangiopancreatography (ERCP)

- Invasive procedure of choice if the bile ducts are not dilated (e.g., sclerosing cholangitis) and if the patient has abnormal bleeding parameters
- Permits therapeutic procedures such as sphincterotomy, stone extraction, brush biopsy of strictures, and insertion of an endoprosthesis

Note: Local experience often dictates the choice between MRCP and ERCP.

 Caveat: Although dilated bile ducts are virtually pathognomonic of extrahepatic biliary obstruction, normal bile ducts do not absolutely exclude this diagnosis because of the underlying disease process (e.g., sclerosing cholangitis) or because the obstruction may be recent or intermittent.

Nausea and Vomiting

Common Causes

Drug reaction (chemotherapeutic agents, central nervous system [CNS]-active drugs, analgesics, cardiovascular drugs, hormones, antibiotics, diuretics, antiasthmatics)

Gastrointestinal disorders

Gastric outlet obstruction (peptic ulcer disease, gastric malignancy, extrinsic compression)

Small bowel obstruction (adhesions, inflammatory bowel disease, neoplasm)

Inflammatory conditions (gastroenteritis, peptic ulcer disease, cholecystitis, pancreatitis, Crohn's disease)

Motility disorders (gastroparesis, irritable bowel syndrome, chronic intestinal pseudoobstruction, scleroderma)

CNS disorders (stroke, neoplasm, labyrinthine disease, motion sickness, psychiatric disorders)

Metabolic conditions (pregnancy, uremia, hyperglycemia, hyperparathyroidism, metabolic acidosis, adrenal insufficiency)

Infectious disorders (hepatitis, meningitis, labyrinthitis)

Approach to Diagnostic Imaging

 Caveat: Initially, a detailed history, physical examination, and laboratory workup should be performed. Appropriate imaging studies can then be ordered, based on the probable clinical diagnosis.

SUSPECTED *GASTROINTESTINAL* CAUSE

■ 1. Plain abdominal radiograph

- Inexpensive initial imaging procedure for detecting a suspected gastric outlet or small bowel obstruction

■ 2. Computed tomography

- Best study for detecting a suspected intra-abdominal inflammatory process (and for further evaluation of small bowel obstruction suggested on plain radiographs)

Peritonitis

Presenting Signs and Symptoms

Generalized abdominal tenderness with rigidity
Absence of bowel sounds
Fever
Vomiting

Common Causes

Perforation of a viscus
Trauma
Strangulating intestinal obstruction
Pancreatitis
Pelvic inflammatory disease
Vascular catastrophe (mesenteric thrombosis or embolus)
Ascites (spontaneous infection or peritoneosystemic shunt)

Approach to Diagnostic Imaging

■ 1. Plain abdominal radiograph

- *Upright* images to demonstrate free air beneath the diaphragm, indicating perforation of a viscus
- If the patient cannot stand or sit, a *lateral decubitus* image (using a horizontal x-ray beam) with the patient's *left* side down may be used (any free air can be more easily detected over the soft-tissue-density liver on the right than when it is overlying luminal air in the stomach, small bowel, or splenic flexure on the left)
- On *supine* images, look for the *double-wall sign* (air outlining both the inner and outer walls of bowel loops), as well as free air outlining the normally invisible falciform and various pelvic ligaments

 Caveat: *NEVER* use barium in the presence of free air in the peritoneal cavity.

■ 2. Computed tomography

- Procedure of choice for detecting loculated fluid collections, abscesses, adynamic ileus, and any type of obstruction including strangulating obstruction

Suspected Abdominal Abscess (No Localized Findings)

Presenting Signs and Symptoms

Spiking fever, chills
Leukocytosis
Indolent course in immunosuppressed patients

Common Causes

Recent surgery or trauma
Alcoholism
Parenteral drug use
Chronic illness
Steroids, chemotherapy, immunosuppressive therapy

Approach to Diagnostic Imaging

■ 1. Computed tomography

- Preferred initial imaging procedure for detecting, characterizing, and determining the extent of an abdominal abscess
- Does not have the disadvantage of the substantial delay required with radionuclide scanning
- Limited value in patients with abrupt and extreme changes in density (metallic clips, residual barium) because of "streak" artifacts

■ 2. Radionuclide scan (indium)

- Can examine the entire abdomen simultaneously and detect multiple or extra-abdominal sites of infection
- Indium is superior to gallium because the normal accumulation of gallium in the liver, spleen, and colon can obscure an abscess. Gallium (but not indium) can accumulate in lymphoma and other neoplasms.

 Caveat: There is a substantial delay before diagnostic results can be obtained (at least 18–24 h after radionuclide injection).

■ 3. Ultrasound

- Alternative to CT in very sick patients (who can only briefly suspend respiration or who cannot leave the intensive care unit)
- Multiplicity of scanning planes may be of value in assessing the precise anatomic relationships of a lesion
- Procedure of choice for children (uses no ionizing radiation)
- Because the examination requires close contact between the transducer and the skin, it may be difficult to perform this test on postsurgical patients with recent incisions, wound dressings, drains, superficial infections, or stomas

Hepatic Abscess

Presenting Signs and Symptoms

Subacute onset of fever, chills, nausea, anorexia, weight loss

Right upper quadrant pain

Hepatomegaly (acute onset suggests multiple abscesses from systemic bacteremia or biliary tract infection)

Common Causes

Ascending cholangitis in a partially or completely obstructed biliary tract

Portal bacteremia from an intraabdominal site (e.g., appendicitis, diverticulitis)

Systemic bacteremia (organisms reach liver through the hepatic artery)

Direct extension from adjacent extrabiliary site

Trauma

Approach to Diagnostic Imaging

■ 1. Computed tomography

- Preferred study for detecting and characterizing a hepatic abscess

■ 2. Ultrasound

- Alternative imaging technique (limited in obese patients) in acutely ill patients who cannot leave the intensive care unit

■ 3. Magnetic resonance imaging

- Indicated in patients who cannot receive iodinated contrast material

Left Subphrenic Space Abscess

Presenting Signs and Symptoms

Left upper quadrant pain and tenderness
Fever
Leukocytosis (increase white cell count)
History of surgery 3–6 weeks before onset

Common Causes

Surgery or trauma
Peritonitis (e.g., perforated viscus)
Spread from distant abdominal abscess

Approach to Diagnostic Imaging

■ 1. Computed tomography

- Preferred initial imaging study (negative CT scan excludes a left subphrenic abscess)
- Ultrasound is usually less effective because of gas in the stomach, small bowel, or colon

■ 2. Radionuclide scan (indium or gallium)

- Indicated if CT is equivocal (not uncommon if there has been recent surgery or trauma) and if it is impossible to differentiate an infected from a sterile collection (e.g., perisplenic hematoma)

 Caveat: Barium studies are contraindicated because retained barium within the bowel significantly delays the performance of more sensitive and specific studies such as CT and radionuclide scans.

Pancreas/Lesser Sac Abscess

Presenting Signs and Symptoms

Fever and abdominal pain arising 10–21 days after acute pancreatitis

Nausea and vomiting

Abdominal mass

Leukocytosis

Increased serum amylase

Approach to Diagnostic Imaging

■ 1. Computed tomography

- Preferred imaging technique
- US is generally ineffective because of the large amounts of intestinal gas related to the usually associated adynamic ileus

Perihepatic Abscess

Presenting Signs and Symptoms

Right upper quadrant pain and tenderness
Fever
Leukocytosis

Common Causes

Prior surgery or trauma

Approach to Diagnostic Imaging

■ 1. Plain abdominal radiograph

- Can detect subtle perihepatic gas collections
- Localized ileus of the hepatic flexure and right pleural effusion are both suggestive but not diagnostic signs, since they may merely reflect nonspecific postoperative or post-traumatic changes

■ 2. Computed tomography

- Preferred imaging technique

■ 3. Ultrasound

- Alternative imaging technique (limited in obese individuals)

■ 4. Radionuclide scan (indium or gallium)

- Examination of the entire abdomen and pelvis is indicated if an occult abscess is still suspected clinically despite negative US and CT studies
- Negative indium or gallium radionuclide scan effectively excludes an abscess

Pelvic Abscess

Presenting Signs and Symptoms

Lower abdominal pain and tenderness
Palpable mass on vaginal or rectal examination
Fever and leukocytosis

Common Causes

Acute appendicitis
Pelvic inflammatory disease
Colon diverticulitis

Approach to Diagnostic Imaging

■ 1. Ultrasound

- Preferred imaging technique for pelvic inflammatory disease
- Fluid-filled urinary bladder provides an excellent acoustic window for examining the supravesical and paravesical spaces

■ 2. Computed tomography

- Preferred initial imaging procedure for men and for women following total abdominal hysterectomy and bilateral salpingo-oophorectomy, as well as for diagnosing perirectal abscesses

■ 3. Magnetic resonance imaging

- Can frequently best define perirectal abscesses and fistulas

■ 4. Radionuclide scan

- May be necessary to confirm the inflammatory nature of the lesion because the differential diagnosis of cystic masses is extensive

 Caveat: Indium is the preferred radionuclide because gallium normally accumulates in the sigmoid and rectum.

Renal/Perirenal Abscess

Presenting Signs and Symptoms

Acute onset of unilateral flank or abdominal pain and
tenderness

Dysuria

Fever, chills

Leukocytosis

Common Cause

Pyelonephritis (often associated with renal calculous
disease, recent urologic surgery, or obstruction by
malignancy)

Approach to Diagnostic Imaging

■ 1. Computed tomography

- Preferred initial imaging technique for detecting
  inflammatory and infectious renal disease
- May demonstrate thickening of Gerota's fascia,
  a subtle change that may be the first sign of a
  perirenal infection

■ 2. Magnetic resonance imaging

- Alternate imaging technique in patients who
  cannot receive iodinated contrast material

■ 3. Ultrasound

- Alternative imaging technique that demonstrates
  a fluid-filled intrarenal or perirenal collection
- Color power Doppler may show abnormal flow
  to infected regions of the kidney

Splenic Abscess

Presenting Signs and Symptoms

Subacute onset of left-sided pain (often pleuritic) in the flank, upper abdomen, or lower chest that may radiate to the left shoulder

Left upper quadrant tenderness

Splenomegaly

Fever

Leukocytosis

Common Causes

Systemic bacteremia (e.g., endocarditis, salmonellosis)

Trauma (superinfection of hematoma)

Extension from contiguous infection (e.g., subphrenic abscess)

Approach to Diagnostic Imaging

■ 1. Computed tomography

- Preferred imaging technique
- US is of less value because most of the spleen lies between the ribs and is largely hidden from the US beam
- MRI is indicated if the patient cannot receive iodinated intravenous contrast material

■ 2. Radionuclide scan (indium or gallium)

- Can specifically identify an intrasplenic mass as an abscess

Abdominal Mass in a Neonate

Organ of Origin

Kidney

Gastrointestinal tract

Approach to Diagnostic Imaging

■ 1. Plain abdominal radiograph

- To exclude obstruction of the gastrointestinal tract

■ 2. Ultrasound

- Can detect intrinsic renal masses and hydrone-phrosis
- If US is normal, no further imaging is required
- If US detects a mass, further imaging depends on the anatomic location and sonographic characteristics of the lesion

■ 3. Magnetic resonance imaging

- Problem-solving modality if ultrasound cannot provide the desired information (requires general anesthesia)

Abdominal Mass in a Child

Organ of Origin

Kidney
Adrenal glands
Pelvic structure

Approach to Diagnostic Imaging

■ 1. Plain abdominal radiograph

- Can detect characteristic calcification associated with neuroblastoma (and its metastases)

■ 2. Ultrasound

- Best initial imaging modality for detecting masses in the kidney, adrenal gland, or genital organs in a child (uses no ionizing radiation)
- Can detect appendiceal abscesses or hepatobiliary lesions, the most common causes of gastrointestinal masses that develop after the neonatal period

■ 3. Cystourethrography

- If US shows a cystic renal mass or severe hydronephrosis, this study can define the bladder anatomy and confirm or exclude vesicoureteral reflux

■ 4. Computed tomography

- Indicated if US shows a solid mass suggestive of malignancy (to better define the anatomy and any local or metastatic spread). It also evaluates kidney function.

Diffusely Enlarged Abdomen (No Discrete Mass)

Common Causes

Ascites
Lipodystrophy
Massive peritoneal/retroperitoneal tumor

Approach to Diagnostic Imaging

■ 1. Computed tomography

- Best modality for defining the organ of origin of any mass in the peritoneal or retroperitoneal compartments
- In patients with massive ascites, can suggest the origin of the peritoneal fluid by detecting masses, metastases, loculation, and the relative distribution of fluid in the lesser and greater sacs
- Adequate US examination is often prevented by gas contained within the stomach, small bowel, and colon

■ 2. Magnetic resonance imaging

- Indicated if the patient cannot receive iodinated intravenous contrast material

Epigastric Mass

Organ of Origin

Liver
Spleen
Stomach
Duodenum
Pancreas

Approach to Diagnostic Imaging

■ 1. Computed tomography

- Directly images the liver, spleen, gastric wall, and pancreas
- Adequate US examination is often prevented by gas contained within the stomach, small bowel, and colon

■ 2. Upper gastrointestinal series

- If there is evidence of gastric outlet obstruction, can evaluate for peptic ulcer or gastric malignancy

■ 3. Magnetic resonance imaging

- Indicated if the patient cannot receive iodinated intravenous contrast material

Hypogastric Mass

Organ of Origin

Bladder
Colon
Uterus
Ovary

Approach to Diagnostic Imaging

■ 1. Ultrasound

- Preferred initial imaging technique because most masses in this region are related to the pelvic organs

■ 2. Computed tomography

- Indicated to better define the extent of a lesion if a solid mass is detected by US

■ 3. Magnetic resonance imaging

- Like US, MRI has no ionizing radiation and is more precise in studying the pelvis.
- Much higher soft-tissue contrast resolution than CT
- Spectroscopic imaging is of value for assessing cancer of the prostate

Left Lower Quadrant Mass

Organ of Origin

Colon

Approach to Diagnostic Imaging

■ 1. Plain abdominal radiograph

- Can demonstrate large bowel obstruction or fecal impaction

■ 2. Computed tomography

- Preferred initial imaging technique for detecting and defining the origin of a palpable mass or the extent of diverticulitis

■ 3. Magnetic resonance imaging

- Indicated if the patient cannot receive iodinated intravenous contrast material

Left Upper Quadrant Mass

Organ of Origin

Spleen
Left lobe of the liver
Stomach (gastric outlet obstruction or tumor)
Splenic flexure of the colon
Pancreas
Left kidney
Left adrenal gland

Approach to Diagnostic Imaging

■ 1. Computed tomography

- Directly images the spleen, liver, gastric wall, pancreas, left kidney, and left adrenal gland
- Adequate US examination is often precluded by gas contained within the stomach, small bowel, and colon

■ 2. Upper gastrointestinal series

- If there is evidence of gastric outlet obstruction, can evaluate for peptic ulcer or gastric malignancy

■ 3. Magnetic resonance imaging

- Indicated if the patient cannot receive iodinated intravenous contrast material

Midabdominal Mass

Organ of Origin

Superficial structures
Peritoneal structures
Retroperitoneal structures

Approach to Diagnostic Imaging

■ 1. Computed tomography

- Directly images the organs within all three compartments
- Adequate US examination is often prevented by gas contained within the stomach, small bowel, and colon

■ 2. Ultrasound

- Initial modality of choice in an asthenic patient with a pulsating mass suggesting aortic aneurysm

■ 3. Magnetic resonance imaging

- Indicated if the patient cannot receive iodinated intravenous contrast material

Right Lower Quadrant Mass

Organ of Origin

Gastrointestinal tract
Abscess
Enlarged lymph nodes

Approach to Diagnostic Imaging

■ 1. Plain abdominal radiograph

- Can exclude or confirm bowel obstruction, appendicolith, or fecal impaction

■ 2. Computed tomography

- Can differentiate among such entities as inflammatory bowel disease, abscess, and enlarged lymph nodes

■ 3. Magnetic resonance imaging

- Indicated if the patient cannot receive iodinated intravenous contrast material

Right Upper Quadrant Mass

Organ of Origin

Right lobe of the liver
Gallbladder
Bile ducts
Right kidney
Right adrenal gland
Hepatic flexure of the colon
Duodenum

Approach to Diagnostic Imaging

■ 1. Ultrasound

- High accuracy for detecting masses involving the gallbladder (acute cholecystitis, hydrops, carcinoma, Courvoisier gallbladder) and bile ducts, as well as diffuse and focal hepatic abnormalities
- Good imaging test for detecting renal lesions and differentiating renal cysts from solid tumors or abscesses

■ 2. Computed tomography

- Indicated if there is bile duct dilatation and US fails to show an obstructing mass
- Indicated for confirmation and staging if US shows a solid renal mass
- Best modality for detecting adrenal masses (metastases, adenoma, carcinoma)

■ 3. Magnetic resonance imaging

- Indicated if the patient cannot receive iodinated intravenous contrast material

Achalasia

Presenting Signs and Symptoms

Dysphagia for solids and liquids (typically in persons 20–40 years old)

Nocturnal regurgitation of undigested food

Aspiration (and recurrent pneumonia)

Common Causes

Primary (idiopathic)

Malignancy (primary or metastatic)

Central and peripheral neuropathy

Cerebrovascular accident

Postvagotomy syndrome

Chagas disease

Approach to Diagnostic Imaging

■ 1. Plain chest radiograph

- ■ Not sensitive, but may demonstrate characteristic findings such as an absent gastric air bubble and an esophageal air–fluid level (best seen in lateral view)

■ 2. Barium swallow

- Dilated esophagus with distal "beak" or "rat-tail" narrowing and an esophageal air–fluid level
- Absence of the gastric air bubble
- Delayed images can assess severity of process

■ 3. Manometry

- Incomplete relaxation of the lower esophageal sphincter
- Absent peristalsis in the smooth-muscle portion of the esophagus

Cancer of the Esophagus

Presenting Signs and Symptoms

Progressive dysphagia (first with solids, then liquids)
Pain (substernal or in the back due to local invasion)
Rapid weight loss
Pulmonary aspiration
Chronic reflux

Risk Factors

Ethanol abuse
Smoking
Barrett's mucosa
Lye ingestion and esophageal stricture
Radiation exposure
Head and neck cancer
Achalasia
Scleroderma
Tylosis
Sprue

Approach to Diagnostic Imaging

■ 1. Barium swallow

- Preferred initial imaging examination that can detect superficial and early (small) tumors if the double-contrast technique is employed
- Cannot identify carcinoma in situ

■ 2. Esophagoscopy (with biopsy and cytology)

- Most sensitive and specific test

Staging

■ 1. Computed tomography (chest/upper abdomen)

- Most effective staging procedure that can determine the potential surgical curability of an esophageal tumor in about 90% of patients
- Accuracy of 97% for detecting tracheobronchial invasion and 94% for aortic and pericardial invasion
- Demonstration of enlarged mediastinal or subdiaphragmatic lymph nodes is likely to represent involvement by metastatic tumor, although the absence of lymphadenopathy is an unreliable finding (since normal-sized nodes also may harbor metastases)

■ 2. Endoscopic ultrasound

- Superior to CT for evaluating the depth of tumor infiltration within the wall of the esophagus (local invasion) and lymph node involvement

Note: US is not as effective as CT in assessing the extra-esophageal spread of tumor, which relates directly to the duration of survival.

■ 3. Positron emission tomography (PET/CT)

- If available, the best preoperative study to evaluate metastatic nodes and distant metastases (better than CT alone)

Diffuse Esophageal Spasm

Presenting Signs and Symptoms

Intermittent substernal chest pain

Dysphagia for both liquids and solids

Symptoms frequently aggravated by very hot or cold liquids

Approach to Diagnostic Imaging

■ 1. Barium swallow

- "Corkscrew" esophagus, sometimes with pseudo-diverticula

■ 2. Manometry

- Most sensitive and specific description of the spasms
- High-amplitude esophageal contractions of long duration with repetitive occurrence

Esophageal Mucosal Laceration (Mallory–Weiss Syndrome)

Presenting Signs and Symptoms

Repeated vomiting followed by hematemesis (especially in men older than age 50 with history of alcohol abuse)

Approach to Diagnostic Imaging

■ 1. Endoscopy

- Required to demonstrate the superficial lacerations or fissures near the esophagogastric junction (usually not seen on radiographic contrast studies)

Note: In rare cases, an esophagram shows contrast penetration into the wall of the esophagus.

Esophageal Perforation

Presenting Signs and Symptoms

Sudden epigastric pain radiating to the shoulder blades after vomiting, retching, or even hiccups (especially after heavy drinking)

Gravely ill appearance with pallor, sweating, tachycardia, and often shock

Common Causes

Boerhaave's syndrome

Penetrating trauma

Complication of endoscopy

Approach to Diagnostic Imaging

■ 1. Plain chest radiograph

- Initial imaging study for detecting air dissecting within the mediastinum and soft tissues, often with pleural effusion or hydropneumothorax

■ 2. Barium swallow

- May demonstrate extravasation through a transmural perforation

 Caveat: *Water-soluble* contrast material must be used first (since barium cannot be cleared from the mediastinum); if the patient cannot protect the airway, use iso-osmolar, non-ionic oral contrast material. If no gross extravasation is shown, use barium (a better contrast agent) to exclude a small leak.

■ 3. Computed tomography

- Preferred study for defining the extent of an inflammatory process in the mediastinum secondary to an esophageal perforation

Reflux Esophagitis

Presenting Signs and Symptoms

Heartburn
Dysphagia (due to stricture)
Upper gastrointestinal bleeding (due to esophageal
ulceration)

Approach to Diagnostic Imaging

■ 1. Upper gastrointestinal series

- Double-contrast examination with magnification
  is often highly reliable in experienced hands.

■ 2. Endoscopy (with mucosal biopsy)

- Preferred study in a patient with active bleeding
- Directly detects esophagitis and peptic strictures
- Can show percancerous dysplasia and Barrett's
  esophagus
- May be normal in gastroesophageal reflux

Scleroderma

Presenting Signs and Symptoms

Often asymptomatic

Heartburn and dysphagia (due to reflux esophagitis secondary to incompetence of lower esophageal sphincter)

Approach to Diagnostic Imaging

■ 1. Barium swallow

- Dilated esophagus with absent peristalsis in the distal 2/3 of the esophagus (smooth muscle)
- Widely patent distal esophagus (in the region of the lower esophageal sphincter)

Note: The distal esophagus may be narrowed in chronic disease because of secondary reflux esophagitis. Patients are at very high risk for developing Barrett's esophagus.

■ 2. Manometry

- Aperistalsis (due to atrophy of esophageal smooth muscle)
- Incompetent lower esophageal sphincter (leading to reflux esophagitis and stricture formation)

Varices (Esophageal/Gastric)

Presenting Sign and Symptom

Upper gastrointestinal bleeding

Common Causes

Cirrhosis
Obstruction of the splenic or portal vein (e.g., carcinoma
of the pancreas)
Hepatic vein obstruction

Approach to Diagnostic Imaging

■ **1. Endoscopy**

- Procedure of choice for acute bleeding

■ **2. Computed tomography**

- Multi-detector study with contrast enhancement
  can show the full extent of the varices and often
  demonstrate the cause

■ **3. Barium swallow**

- Can demonstrate characteristic tortuous, beaded
  filling defects in the distal esophagus and
  gastric fundus

Interventional Radiologic Alternative

■ **1. Transjugular intrahepatic portosystemic
shunt (TIPS)**

- Effective and reliable means of lowering portal
  venous pressure (particularly in patients with
  acute variceal bleeding unresponsive to sclero-
  therapy or with chronic variceal bleeding before
  liver transplantation)
- Useful in the treatment of ascites and the Budd-
  Chiari syndrome

Cancer of the Stomach

Presenting Signs and Symptoms

Progressive upper abdominal discomfort
Weight loss, anorexia, nausea, vomiting
Acute or chronic upper gastrointestinal bleeding
Early satiety

Risk Factors

Dietary habits (nitrates, smoked or heavily salted foods)
Atrophic gastritis (pernicious anemia)
H. pylori infection
Billroth II gastroenterostomy (antrectomy with gastro-jejunostomy)
Adenomatous gastric polyps

Approach to Diagnostic Imaging

■ 1. Upper gastrointestinal series

- Preferred initial radiologic imaging procedure
- Requires meticulous technique to detect small, early lesions

■ 2. Endoscopy (with biopsy and cytology)

- Most sensitive and specific test (sensitivity of up to 98% if multiple biopsy specimens are taken from a suspicious lesion to decrease the risk of sampling error)

Staging

■ 1. Computed tomography

- Most effective staging procedure for demonstrating the presence and extent of extragastric spread of tumor
- More accurate in detecting distant lymphadenopathy than local lymph node enlargement

■ 2. Positron emission tomography (PET/CT)

- Better than CT alone for detecting metastatic nodes

■ 3. Endoscopic ultrasound (EUS)

- Good for assessing the depth of mural invasion (T stage) and the status of local lymph nodes (N stage)

Peptic Ulcer Disease

Presenting Signs and Symptoms

Burning epigastric pain (90–180 min after meals, often nocturnal, relieved by food)

Chronic, recurring course

Gastrointestinal bleeding (melena, hematemesis, hematochezia)

Gastric outlet obstruction (about 5%)

Acute abdomen (if free perforation)

Approach to Diagnostic Imaging

■ 1. Upper gastrointestinal series

- Signs of benignity include a smooth ulcer mound with tapering edges, an edematous ulcer collar with overhanging mucosal edge, projection of the ulcer beyond the expected lumen, a blood clot within the ulcer crater, and thin radiating folds extending into the crater

- Size, depth, number, and location of the ulcer are of no diagnostic value in differentiating benign from malignant (except for ulcers in the cardia and gastric fundus, which are virtually always malignant). With the double-contrast technique, excellent coasting of the mucosa and good distension of the stomach, gastric erosions can be seen.

■ 2. Endoscopy

- May be preferable for suspected gastric ulcer, since biopsy can be performed to exclude malignancy
- More reliable for detecting acute ulcer craters in a scarred duodenum
- Fails to detect 5–10% of peptic ulcers

 Caveat: Once the diagnosis of benign peptic disease has been made, recurrences should be treated symptomatically; there is *no* need to repeat an imaging procedure with each recurrence.

Zollinger–Ellison Syndrome

Presenting Signs and Symptoms

Refractory peptic ulcer disease (after medical therapy or surgery)
Gastric hypersecretion
Diarrhea
Substantially elevated serum gastrin

Common Cause

Gastrinoma (usually of the pancreas)

Approach to Diagnostic Imaging

■ 1. Computed tomography

- Preferred study for detecting the underlying pancreatic tumor, which typically is small, often multiple, and intensely enhancing

■ 2. Magnetic resonance imaging

- Contrast-enhanced MRI has become an excellent alternative to CT, particularly in patients who cannot received iodinated contrast material

■ 3. Upper gastrointestinal series

- May show characteristic pattern of markedly thickened gastric folds and ulcers distal to the duodenal bulb (seen in about half the patients), gastric hypersecretion, and enlarged folds.

Pyloric Stenosis

Presenting Signs and Symptoms

Projectile, nonbilious vomiting
Typically occurs in 2- to 6-week-old males
Palpable midabdominal mass ("pyloric olive")

Approach to Diagnostic Imaging

■ 1. Ultrasound

- Preferred imaging technique with almost 100% sensitivity
- Demonstrates characteristic "doughnut" or "target" lesion (hypoechoic wall surrounding echogenic mucosa) on transverse view and elongated pyloric channel on longitudinal scan

■ 2. Upper gastrointestinal series

- Indicated if US is negative and vomiting persists

Small Bowel Obstruction

Presenting Signs and Symptoms

Crampy abdominal pain and bloating
Nausea and vomiting
Abdominal tenderness and peritoneal signs
Abdominal distension
Increased high-pitched bowel sounds

Common Causes

Adhesions
Hernia
Tumor
Intussusception
Extrinsic mass

Approach to Diagnostic Imaging

■ 1. Plain abdominal radiograph

- Change in caliber of air-filled bowel (dilated proximally, collapsed distally)
- String-of-beads sign on upright films

■ 2. Computed tomography

- Much more accurate than small bowel follow-through with oral contrast agent for demonstrating the underlying cause of the obstruction

 Caveat: If CT scan is inconclusive and an oral contrast examination is needed to confirm an obstruction, use barium, *NOT* water-soluble agents, for small bowel follow-through (hyperosmolar contrast draws fluid into the bowel, diluting the opaque material and making it difficult to clearly show the site of obstruction). Before barium is given by mouth, it is necessary to exclude a large bowel obstruction (use water-soluble contrast).

Intussusception

Presenting Signs and Symptoms

CHILDREN

Colicky abdominal pain that waxes and wanes

Vomiting, diarrhea, and other gastrointestinal symptoms in greater than 90% of patients

Palpable abdominal mass in about 50% of patients

Heme-positive or "currant jelly" stools

Accounts for 80–90% of bowel obstruction in infants and children

Peak incidence at 3–9 months (40%); 50% of cases occur at less than 1 year and 75% at less than 2 years; only 10% occur after age 3

ADULTS

General signs and symptoms of bowel obstruction

Often chronic and relapsing (diagnosis suggested by recurrent episodes of subacute obstruction and by variability of abdominal signs)

Palpable mass may be present during the height of an attack and disappear completely when the patient is reexamined several hours later, by which time the symptoms have resolved

Combination of an abdominal mass and the passage of blood per rectum suggests the diagnosis

Common Causes

CHILDREN

Idiopathic in 95% (most commonly involves ileocolic region); mucosal edema and lymphoid hyperplasia often follow viral gastroenteritis

Lead point in 5% (may be Meckel's diverticulum, lymphoma, duplication cyst, enterogenous cyst, inspissated meconium, Henoch-Schönlein purpura)

ADULTS

Specific cause in 80% (benign tumor in 33%, malignant tumor in 20%; also Meckel's diverticulum, adhesions, sprue, scleroderma)

Idiopathic in 20%

Approach to Diagnostic Imaging

■ 1. Plain abdominal radiograph

- Normal in 25%
- Small bowel obstruction in 25%
- Abdominal soft-tissue mass highlighted by bowel gas (crescent sign)

■ 2. Contrast enema

- Characteristic "coiled-spring" appearance
- Abrupt, beak-like narrowing of the contrast column demonstrating a central channel
- Barium enema can be employed both diagnostically and therapeutically in a medically stable child. Surgical consultation is needed prior to the study in case reduction is unsuccessful or a complication occurs.
- Water-soluble contrast or air can also be employed both diagnostically and therapeutically

 Caveat: Reduction of an intussusception should *not* be attempted in adults.

■ 3. Ultrasound

- Shows a target or doughnut appearance on transverse scans and a "pseudokidney" sign on longitudinal scans
- Most useful when the clinical suspicion is low and there is reluctance to perform a barium enema, or when a child is extremely ill and surgery is contemplated

 Caveat: US is *not* recommended in adults.

■ 4. Computed tomography

- Used when evaluating a patient for suspected small bowel obstruction
- May demonstrate a target sign, a sausage-shaped mass with alternating areas of low and high attenuation, or a reniform mass

Gastroenteritis

Presenting Signs and Symptoms

Anorexia, nausea, vomiting
Diarrhea of variable severity
Abdominal discomfort
Low-grade fever
Travel history

Common Causes

Bacterial, viral, or parasitic infection
Enterotoxins (bacterial)
Chemical toxins (mushrooms, shellfish, contaminated food)
Food allergies

Approach to Diagnostic Imaging

No imaging studies are required unless examinations of stool specimens and stool cultures are negative and symptoms persist

Meckel's Diverticulum

Presenting Signs and Symptoms

Rectal bleeding (ulcerating gastric mucosa within a diverticulum)

Bowel obstruction

Common Cause

Omphalomesenteric duct remnant in distal small bowel within 100 cm of ileocecal valve

Approach to Diagnostic Imaging

■ 1. Radionuclide scan (technetium)

- Focal right lower quadrant accumulation of isotope by gastric mucosa lining the diverticulum

Antibiotic-Associated Colitis (Pseudomembranous Colitis)

Presenting Signs and Symptoms

Range from transient mild diarrhea to a severe colitis that develops during a course of antibiotic therapy or up to 6 weeks after treatment has ended

Common Causes

Toxin-producing strains of *Clostridium difficile* (growing especially after clindamycin, ampicillin, cephalosporins, or aminoglycosides)

Approach to Diagnostic Imaging

■ 1. Sigmoidoscopy

- Directly shows characteristic pseudomembranes

■ 2. Computed tomography

- Demonstrates mural thickening of a hypodense colon wall
- Because symptoms may be misleading, may suggest the correct diagnosis before it is suspected clinically

Appendicitis

Presenting Signs and Symptoms

Sudden onset of epigastric or periumbilical pain that shifts to the right lower quadrant

Rebound tenderness

Low-grade fever

Leukocytosis

Approach to Diagnostic Imaging

■ 1. Plain abdominal radiograph

- Low sensitivity and specificity, but may detect a calcified appendicolith (about 15%), which is strongly associated with perforation, especially in children

■ 2. Computed tomography

- "Gold standard" for the noninvasive diagnosis of appendicitis
- With contrast enhancement, can make the diagnosis by identifying an abnormal appendix (dilated with a thickened, circumferentially enhancing wall) or pericecal inflammation and/or abscess associated with an appendicolith
- More sensitive than US for revealing the normal appendix, a critical observation, since definitive exclusion of appendicitis requires visualization of the normal appendix in its entirety

Note: Multi-detector CT imaging is increasingly being used as an alternative to sonography for diagnosing possible appendicitis in nonpregnant patients, in grossly obese or large body habitus patients, in patients with severe abdominal pain, and in patients in whom sonography is inconclusive.

- Highly accurate for showing unrelated intra-abdominal disease that may mimic appendicitis and explain the patient's clinical presentation
- Can be used to guide percutaneous abscess drainage
- Detects appendicolith in about 30% of patients

■ 3. Ultrasound

- Highly sensitive and specific without need for ionizing radiation (especially in children and women during childbearing years)
- Disadvantages include high operator dependence and limitations due to obesity, large amounts of intestinal gas, and patients with retrocecal appendix or severe abdominal pain

■ 4. Magnetic resonance imaging

- Has been used with moderate success in pregnant women

Cancer of the Colon

Presenting Signs and Symptoms

Bright red rectal bleeding, altered bowel habits, abdominal or back pain (left-sided lesions)

Iron deficiency anemia, occult blood in the stool, weight loss (right-sided lesions)

Risk Factors

Diet (low in fiber, high in animal fat)
Personal or family history of colorectal polyps
Familial polyposis syndrome
Family history of colorectal cancer
Chronic Ulcerative colitis
Crohn's colitis
Hypercholesterolemia

Approach to Diagnostic Imaging

■ 1. Colonoscopy

- Slightly more sensitive and specific than barium enema, but associated with considerably higher cost and complications
- Provides excellent color images and an opportunity for biopsying lesions
- Blind spots behind folds or around the flexures

■ 2. CT colonoscopy (virtual colonoscopy)

- Increasingly popular examination that is still evolving. Highly accurate when performed by experienced radiologists familiar with the examination, using up-to-date equipment and software and preferably with computer-aided detection (CAD)
- Permits the detection of synchronous lesions proximal to a high-grade obstruction

■ 3. Barium enema

- Now performed primarily in patients who are too sick to undergo colonoscopy or if colonoscopy cannot be successfully performed for some reason.
- This study has fallen out of favor for screening patients at average risk for colorectal cancer, but remains an accurate diagnostic tool when properly performed

Staging

■ 1. Computed tomography

- Most effective staging procedure for demonstrating the presence and extent of extracolonic spread of tumor

■ 2. Transrectal ultrasound

- Most accurate imaging method for staging local rectal cancer (can assess the depth of invasion within the bowel wall and can suggest the presence of tumor in adjacent normal-sized lymph nodes)

■ 3. Magnetic resonance imaging

- Better soft-tissue contrast resolution than CT, but its higher cost and time requirement relegates it to a problem-solving role.
- Superior to CT for staging advanced rectal cancer

■ 4. Positron emission tomography (PET/CT)

- Superior to CT alone for detection of metastatic lymph nodes and liver metastases

Screening

Indications for screening

General population: after age 50, every 5 years by either
Colonoscopy
CT colonography (virtual colonoscopy)

Positive family history or genetic screening: after age
30, every 2 years

Familial adenomatous polyposis: yearly colonoscopy
beginning at puberty; a colectomy with ileo-anal
pouch reconstruction is usually performed in the
late teenage years or early 20s

Ulcerative colitis and Crohn's colitis: annually after
5–10 years of disease

Note: CT colonography (virtual colonoscopy) has evolved
into an excellent screening approach. However, it needs
experienced examiners, modern equipment and software,
and computer-aided detection (CAD). It is expensive and
at present needs extensive bowel cleansing, which must be
repeated if biopsy or removal of polyps is required. New
approaches with barium ingestion and low-residue diet
show promise.

Ulcerative Colitis

Presenting Signs and Symptoms

Bloody diarrhea

Mucus in stool

Abdominal pain (ranging from mild lower abdominal cramping to severe peritoneal signs)

Fever

Complications (toxic megacolon, colon perforation, hemorrhage, increased risk of cancer)

Approach to Diagnostic Imaging

■ 1. Sigmoidoscopy

- Direct and immediate indication of the activity of the disease process

■ 2. Plain abdominal radiograph

- To exclude toxic megacolon
- Distal extent of formed fecal residue gives a good indication (although not absolute) of the proximal extent of the colitis (may overestimate but does not underestimate extent of disease)

■ 3. Colonoscopy

- To determine the full extent of the disease and detect the development of malignancy in patients with chronic disease

■ 4. Computed tomography

- Demonstrates edematous thickening of the wall of the colon as well as pericolonic inflammatory changes. The ulcers are too superficial to visualize, unless there is a perforation.

Crohn's Disease

Presenting Signs and Symptoms

Abdominal pain

Fever

Anorexia and weight loss

Diarrhea (often without blood)

Fatigue

Right lower quadrant mass or fullness

Anorectal fissures, fistulas, abscesses (may be acute ileitis mimicking appendicitis or obstruction)

Complications (bowel obstruction, internal fistulas, and bile salt malabsorption leading to gallstones or oxalate kidney stones)

Approach to Diagnostic Imaging

■ 1. Barium enema

- Demonstrates involvement of the terminal ileum and variable amounts of colon and more proximal small bowel disease characterized by nodularity and thickening of folds, aphthoid ulcers, narrowing and rigidity, cobblestoning, string sign, skip areas, and fistulas

■ 2. Small bowel examination

- Required if the terminal ileum is not visualized because of an inability to reflux barium through a competent ileocecal valve

■ 3. Enteroclysis

- Excellent technique, but requires experienced examiners and has patient acceptance only if conscious sedation is used

■ 4. Computed tomography

- In addition to showing thickening of the bowel wall indicating disease activity, the best modality for demonstrating mesenteric and extraintestinal extent of disease and abscess formation

■ 5. CT enteroclysis

- Highly accurate technique combining the advantages of both approaches. However, disadvantages of this complicated procedure include cost, time, and logistics (fluoroscopic positioning of the tube, intravenous contrast, and precise scheduling of CT).

■ 6. MR enteroclysis

- Advantages of no ionizing radiation and exquisite soft-tissue evaluation.

Diverticulitis

Presenting Signs and Symptoms

Abdominal pain and tenderness (typically left lower quadrant)

Altered bowel habits

Fever

Leukocytosis

Approach to Diagnostic Imaging

■ 1. Computed tomography

- Demonstrates pericolonic fluid or a gas collection (abscess), usually with nonspecific thickening of the colon wall, narrowing of the colonic lumen, and inflammatory stranding in adjacent fat
- Can be used to guide percutaneous abscess drainage

■ 2. Barium enema

- May demonstrate extravasation of contrast through a diverticular perforation *or* a pericolic soft-tissue mass (walled-off perforation) causing eccentric narrowing of the colon

 Caveat: If free perforation into the peritoneal cavity is suspected, *water-soluble* contrast must be used.

Note: Plain abdominal radiographs are *not* needed unless there are peritoneal signs suggesting free perforation.

Diverticulosis

Presenting Signs and Symptoms

Often asymptomatic
Unexplained lower gastrointestinal bleeding
Recurrent left lower quadrant pain
Alternating constipation and diarrhea

Approach to Diagnostic Imaging

■ 1. Barium enema

- Contrast-filled outpouchings from the colon without evidence of extravasation or mass effect

 Caveat: It can be extremely difficult to exclude a polyp or carcinoma in a segment of colon that is severely involved by diverticular disease (usually discovered during colonoscopy).

Fecal Incontinence

Presenting Signs and Symptoms

Involuntary passage of stool through the anus

Common Causes

Rectal prolapse

Anorectal trauma

Abnormal rectal compliance (inflammatory bowel disease, radiation proctitis, rectal ischemia)

Irritable bowel syndrome

Polyneuropathies

CNS disorders (dementia, stroke, brain tumor, multiple sclerosis, spinal cord lesion)

Following complicated childbirth

Approach to Diagnostic Imaging

■ 1. Manometry

- Anal manometry is indicated to measure basal and squeeze pressures in the anal canal
- Rectal balloon manometry is performed to measure rectal sensation, rectal compliance, anorectal inhibitory reflex, and anorectal contractile response

■ 2. Defecography

- Assesses the anorectal angle, perineal descent, and puborectalis muscle function

■ 3. Anal endosonography

- Evaluates the integrity of the sphincter

■ 4. Magnetic resonance imaging

- Evaluates the integrity of the sphincter
- Dynamic studies can also depict the pelvic floor

Hemorrhoids

Presenting Signs and Symptoms

Bleeding (typically after defecation and noted on the toilet tissue)

Pain (if ulcerated, thrombosed, or strangulated)

Protrusion (may regress spontaneously or be reduced manually)

Approach to Diagnostic Imaging

Imaging is *not* indicated

Barium enema examination should only be performed if there is clinical evidence of a more serious cause of rectal bleeding (hemorrhoidal bleeding rarely leads to anemia or an acute exsanguinating hemorrhage)

Hirschsprung's Disease

Presenting Signs and Symptoms

Constipation in the first month of life due to absence of ganglion cells in the myenteric plexus of the rectum and distal colon

Approach to Diagnostic Imaging

■ 1. Plain abdominal radiograph

- Demonstrates distal bowel obstruction with a large amount of retained feces and a greatly distended colon

Note: There is *no* indication for an upper gastrointestinal series.

■ 2. Contrast enema

- Shows precise level of colonic obstruction

Note: A normal contrast enema examination does not entirely exclude short-segment Hirschsprung's disease of the anus. An anorectal biopsy may be needed if the index of suspicion remains high.

Irritable Bowel Syndrome

Presenting Signs and Symptoms

Symptoms triggered by stress or ingestion of foods
Pasty, ribbon-like, or pencil-thin stools
Mucus (not blood) in the stools
Onset often before age 30 (especially in women)

Common Variants

Spastic colon (chronic abdominal pain and constipation)
Alternating constipation and diarrhea
Chronic painless diarrhea

Approach to Diagnostic Imaging

■ 1. Barium enema

■ Primarily performed to exclude inflammatory bowel disease or malignancy

Note: Colonoscopy is frequently performed, generally showing normal findings

Large Bowel Obstruction

Presenting Signs and Symptoms

Gradually increasing constipation leading to obstipation and abdominal distension

Lower abdominal cramps unproductive of feces

Vomiting (if incompetent ileocecal valve)

Common Causes

Malignant tumor

Inflammatory stricture (e.g., diverticulitis)

Volvulus

Hernia

Extrinsic lesion

Approach to Diagnostic Imaging

■ 1. Plain abdominal radiograph

- Change in caliber of gas-filled colon at the site of obstruction
- Lateral decubitus view (right side down) can allow gas to rise into the sigmoid and rectum and can differentiate between colonic adynamic ileus (rectum/sigmoid distended) and mechanical obstruction (rectum/sigmoid remain collapsed)

■ 2. Computed tomography

- Especially valuable in patients without a history of surgery who have systemic signs suggesting infection, bowel infarction, or an associated palpable mass
- Can demonstrate diverticulitis or appendicitis as the cause of an obstruction

Note: Some radiologists recommend CT as the initial study (instead of barium enema) as a more direct means for establishing the diagnosis of large bowel obstruction.

■ 3. Barium enema

- Shows site and character of the obstruction.

Notes: In patients with *acute* obstruction, *water-soluble* contrast material should be used (due to the danger of barium inspissation proximal to a colonic obstruction; if there is an adynamic ileus, retained barium will remain for a prolonged period and interfere with other imaging studies).

In patients with intussusception or volvulus, a barium enema may be therapeutic as well as diagnostic.

If endoscopy is to be performed, it should *precede* the barium enema. CT should also precede the barium enema, since residual barium in the large bowel may persist for several days, particularly in elderly patients, and prolong their hospitalization.

Biliary Obstruction

Presenting Signs and Symptoms

Yellowing of skin and sclera (jaundice)
Abnormal liver enzymes
Dark urine and pale, clay-colored stools

Common Causes

Common duct stone
Pancreatic carcinoma
Cholangiocarcinoma
Obstructing metastases

Approach to Diagnostic Imaging

■ 1. Computed tomography or ultrasound

- Demonstrates bile duct dilatation indicative of obstruction
- CT is highly accurate for showing disease in adjacent structures (liver, porta hepatis, pancreas, adrenals, retroperitoneum)
- Neither CT nor US can reliably exclude a common duct stone (sensitivity less than 80–85%), but no further imaging tests are needed when choledocholithiasis is diagnosed by these modalities

■ 2. Magnetic resonance cholangiopancreatography (MRCP)

- Preferred non-invasive approach if CT and US do not prove conclusive

■ 3. Endoscopic retrograde cholangiopancreatography (ERCP)

- Invasive procedure of choice if the bile ducts are not dilated (e.g., sclerosing cholangitis) and if the patient has abnormal bleeding parameters
- Permits therapeutic procedures (e.g., sphincter-otomy, stone extraction, brush biopsy of strictures, and insertion of an endoprosthesis) at the time of initial diagnosis
- Highly operator-dependent (unsuccessful duct cannulation in 3–9% of patients) and substantial morbidity and mortality (7% and 1%, respectively)
- Limited or no opacification of ducts proximal to a severe or complete obstruction
- Routine sedation required

Cholecystitis (Acute)

Presenting Signs and Symptoms

Acute colicky right upper quadrant pain and tenderness
Fever
Nausea and vomiting
Mild jaundice (occasionally)
Mild leukocytosis
Mild elevation of serum bilirubin, alkaline phosphatase, and serum glutamic oxaloacetic transaminase (SGOT)

Approach to Diagnostic Imaging

■ 1. Ultrasound

- May demonstrate gallstones, thickening of the gallbladder wall, pericholecystic fluid, and point tenderness directly over the gallbladder (sonographic Murphy's sign)
- Permits detection of abnormalities of the liver, pancreas, or kidneys that may produce a clinical appearance mimicking acute cholecystitis (only about one-third of patients with symptoms of acute cholecystitis actually have that condition)
- Indicated if there is strong clinical evidence of acalculous nonobstructing acute cholecystitis in the face of a negative cholescintigram

■ 2. Cholescintigraphy (technetium-IDA derivatives)

- Visualized gallbladder *excludes* acute cholecystitis (specificity 95%) by indicating patency of the cystic duct
- Nonvisualized gallbladder after 4h strongly *suggests* acute cholecystitis (sensitivity 98%) if the patient is not a chronic alcoholic or undergoing total parenteral nutrition

---

Note: With the use of morphine augmentation, the time required to perform a radionuclide study is reduced to 1.5h.

■ 3. Magnetic resonance cholangiopancreatography (MRCP)

- Indicated when US findings are not diagnostic
- US is superior to MRCP for evaluating gallbladder wall thickness, but MRCP is better for depicting the cystic duct and obstructing calculi in the gallbladder neck

Cholecystitis (Chronic)

Presenting Signs and Symptoms

Recurrent right upper quadrant pain and biliary colic

Approach to Diagnostic Imaging

■ 1. Ultrasound

- Preferred initial imaging technique
- Demonstrates high-amplitude echo in the gall-bladder lumen (reflecting from the surface of a gallstone) or in the gallbladder fossa (if the lumen is completely filled with calculi) associated with posterior acoustic shadowing

■ 2. Cholescintigraphy

- Cholecystokinin (CCK)-enhanced study can evaluate the ejection fraction of the gallbladder, which is diminished in chronic cholecystitis

 Caveat: Plain abdominal radiographs are of limited value, since only about 20% of gallstones are radiopaque.

■ 3. Computed tomography

- Baseline examination to give information about the liver, pancreas, and upper abdomen

Fatty Liver

Presenting Signs and Symptoms

Asymptomatic hepatomegaly

Possible right upper quadrant pain, tenderness, or jaundice

Common Causes

Cirrhosis

Chemicals/drugs (e.g., alcohol, steroids, tetracyclines, carbon tetrachloride, methotrexate)

Obesity

Malnutrition

Hyperalimentation

Cystic fibrosis

Approach to Diagnostic Imaging

■ 1. Computed tomography

- Noncontrast CT demonstrates diffuse low attenuation of the liver parenchyma (lower than that of the spleen)
- Focal fatty infiltration may simulate a liver tumor (although vessels typically run their normal course through the area of involvement)

■ 2. Magnetic resonance imaging

- May be needed to exclude a hepatic mass when focal fat deposition is seen on CT or US in a patient with a malignancy. Fat-suppression techniques are also valuable.

Hemangioma of the Liver

Presenting Signs and Symptoms

Asymptomatic and discovered incidentally on US, CT, or MRI

Approach to Diagnostic Imaging

■ 1. Ultrasound, computed tomography, magnetic resonance imaging, or radionuclide scan

- US may show a typically well-defined, hyper-echoic mass
- CT may demonstrate a low-attenuation mass with well-defined borders on nonenhanced scans; after contrast injection, there may be character-istic filling in of the lesion in a centripetal fash-ion (entire mass becomes isodense). Enhancing areas are isodense with the blood pool.
- MRI may show marked hyperintensity of the mass on T2-weighted images with an enhance-ment pattern similar to that on CT
- Radionuclide scan using tagged red blood cells shows prolonged activity within the lesion on delayed images (preferred imaging study if the lesion is >3 cm)

Notes: If the lesion has a *characteristic* appear-ance, it should be left alone with no further imaging studies.

If the patient has a known malignancy, abnormal liver function tests, or symptoms, *more than one* imaging study should be performed.

Portal Hypertension

Presenting Signs and Symptoms

Bleeding esophageal varices
Ascites and edema
Encephalopathy
Nonspecific constitutional symptoms of fatigue, lethargy, anorexia

Common Causes

Cirrhosis
Obstruction of the extrahepatic portal vein (e.g., carcinoma of the pancreas)
Hepatic vein obstruction

Approach to Diagnostic Imaging

■ 1. Color and duplex Doppler ultrasound

- Demonstrates patency and direction of blood flow in hepatic veins, portal veins, and collateral venous channels

■ 2. Computed tomography

- Documents presence of venous collaterals in the mesentery and retroperitoneum
- Can better define the cause of extrahepatic portal vein thrombosis and any propagation into the liver

■ 3. Magnetic resonance angiography

- Indicated if intravenous contrast material is contraindicated or if CT is inconclusive

Hepatocellular Carcinoma (Hepatoma)

Presenting Signs and Symptoms

Right upper quadrant pain
Tender hepatomegaly
Unexplained deterioration in a previously stable patient with cirrhosis
Weight loss
Fever (may simulate infection)
Elevated serum α-fetoprotein (in 60–90%)

Risk Factors

Chronic hepatitis B infection
Cirrhosis (especially alcohol-induced)
Hemochromatosis
Thorotrast exposure (radiographic contrast agent used from about 1940 to 1960)

Approach to Diagnostic Imaging

■ 1. Computed tomography

- Preferred initial imaging technique for demonstrating any of the three major patterns (diffuse infiltrative, solitary massive, and multinodular)
- Multiphasic MDCT scanning (including hepatic arterial phase) is needed to establish the diagnosis of this vascular tumor

■ 2. Magnetic resonance imaging

- May permit a specific diagnosis of hepatocellular carcinoma by demonstrating
  - (1) characteristic capsule of compressed liver or scar tissue,
  - (2) accumulation of fat within the tumor, and
  - (3) propensity of tumor spread into the hepatic and portal veins
- Should be performed during the arterial phase following gadolinium administration, or even better if dynamic scanning is possible.

■ 3. Ultrasound

- Used in high-prevalence areas (e.g., Japan, Vietnam) for screening of chronic hepatitis B virus carriers. Has been less successful for screening Western populations.

Liver Metastases

Presenting Signs and Symptoms

Usually asymptomatic

May have nonspecific weight loss, anorexia, fever, weakness

Hepatomegaly (hard and often tender)

Ascites

Jaundice

Common Primary Tumors

Gastrointestinal tract (colon, pancreas, stomach)

Lung

Breast

Lymphoma

Melanoma

Approach to Diagnostic Imaging

■ 1. Computed tomography

- Sensitive screening technique that is preferred to MRI if there is also a need to assess possible metastases in the adrenal glands, retroperitoneum, and other abdominal organs
- Permits fine-needle aspiration biopsy for cytology to provide a definitive diagnosis

■ 2. Magnetic resonance imaging

- Sensitive technique for detecting liver metastases
- Generally indicated in patients who cannot receive intravenous iodinated contrast or who are being considered for partial hepatectomy
- Improved sensitivity with the use of contrast agents containing iron or manganese

■ 3. Transabdominal ultrasound

- Less sensitive than MRI, CT, or PET/CT, but is rapid and inexpensive and reliably identifies the majority of patients with hepatic metastases

■ 4. PET/CT

- Combining the functional capabilities of PET and the spatial resolution of CT, this modality can be used to stage patients, especially if planning hepatic resection.

■ 5. Intraoperative ultrasound

- Most sensitive technique for detecting hepatic metastases

 Caveat: Radionuclide scan is less sensitive than other methods for detecting liver metastases and thus is *not* indicated for routine screening.

Pancreatitis (Acute)

Presenting Signs and Symptoms

Steady, boring midepigastric pain radiating straight through to the back

Elevated serum amylase and lipase

Common Causes

Biliary tract disease (e.g., stones)

Alcoholism

Drugs

Infection (e.g., mumps)

Hyperlipidemia

ERCP

Neoplasm

Surgery or trauma

Approach to Diagnostic Imaging

■ 1. Computed tomography

- Imaging procedure of choice for demonstrating focal or diffuse enlargement of the gland and indistinctness of its margins
- Superior to US for showing extrapancreatic spread of inflammation and edema and for detecting gas within a pancreatic fluid collection (highly suggestive of abscess)
- Can also be used to suggest the prognosis

■ 2. Magnetic resonance imaging (with MRCP)

- Useful in staging pancreatitis and detecting stones in the common bile duct and pancreatic duct

■ 3. Ultrasound

- In addition to demonstrating symmetric enlargement of a relatively sonolucent gland, may show cholelithiasis, an important underlying cause of acute pancreatitis
- Frequent occurrence of adynamic ileus with excessive intestinal gas may prevent adequate visualization of the gland
- Useful for follow-up of specific abnormalities (e.g., fluid collections)

 Caveat: Although plain abdominal radiographs are abnormal in 50% of patients, they usually show only generalized or localized ileus that is *not specific* for pancreatitis.

Pancreatitis (Chronic)

Presenting Signs and Symptoms

Midepigastric pain

Weight loss, steatorrhea, and other signs and symptoms of malabsorption

Common Causes

Alcoholism

Hereditary pancreatitis

Hyperparathyroidism

Obstruction of main pancreatic duct (stricture, stones, cancer)

Approach to Diagnostic Imaging

■ 1. Plain abdominal radiograph

- Demonstrates virtually pathognomonic pancreatic calcifications in 30–60% of patients

■ 2. Computed tomography or magnetic resonance imaging (with MRCP)

- Shows enlargement or atrophy of the gland, dilatation of the pancreatic duct, and pseudocyst formation
- CT shows parenchymal and intraductal stones better than MRI

■ 3. Endoscopic retrograde cholangiopancreatography (ERCP)

- Shows irregular dilatation of the main pancreatic duct and pruning of its branches

Cancer of the Pancreas

Presenting Signs and Symptoms

Abdominal and back pain
Weight loss and anorexia
Painless jaundice
Enlarged, palpable gallbladder (Courvoisier's sign)

Approach to Diagnostic Imaging

■ 1. Computed tomography

- Shows a mass with (or without) obstructive dilatation of the pancreatic or bile duct or both
- Most effective modality for demonstrating lesions in the tail and for defining the extent of tumor spread (may prevent needless surgery in patients with nonresectable lesions)

■ 2. Magnetic resonance imaging (with MRCP)

- Can provide one-stop evaluation of pancreatic cancer: diagnosis; staging; vascular and ductal assessment

■ 3. Endoscopic retrograde cholangiopancreatography (ERCP)

- Most sensitive test for tumors of the pancreatic head (deformity/stricture of the bile duct)
- Indicated if clinical suspicion remains high in the face of normal CT and MR examinations

Interventional Radiologic Alternatives

■ 1. Percutaneous fine-needle aspiration (under CT or US guidance)

- Often provides a precise histologic diagnosis

■ 2. Percutaneous stent placement for biliary drainage

- May be performed using either ERCP or PTHC

Trauma (Blunt Abdominal)

Approach to Diagnostic Imaging

■ 1. Plain abdominal and chest radiographs

- Neither sensitive nor specific, but inexpensive and rapidly available. Can direct attention to specific organ injuries

  - ■ SPLEEN
    - Fractures of lower left ribs
    - Elevation of left hemidiaphragm
    - Left pleural effusion
    - Displacement of gastric air bubble
    - Irregular splenic outline

  - ■ LIVER
    - Fractures of right lower ribs
    - Displacement of hepatic flexure
    - Irregular/enlarged hepatic outline

  - ■ RETROPERITONEUM
    - Loss of psoas or renal shadow
    - Free retroperitoneal gas
    - Fracture of lumbar transverse process

  - ■ DIAPHRAGM
    - Herniation of abdominal contents into chest
    - Abnormal position of nasogastric tube
    - Elevation and loss of definition of hemi-diaphragm
    - Nonspecific pleural effusion and atelectasis

■ 2. Computed tomography

- Highest sensitivity and specificity for detecting injuries to the liver, spleen, kidneys, and retro-peritoneum

■ 3. Radionuclide scan or ultrasound

- Only indicated if CT examination of the liver and spleen is ambiguous because of surgical clip artifacts or motion (or if an allergy to intravenous contrast precludes an enhanced CT study)

■ 4. Arteriography

- Only indicated if both CT and radionuclide scan are equivocal (especially valuable as both a diagnostic and therapeutic tool in patients with pelvic ring disruption who have evidence of severe bleeding)

 Caveat: Although diagnostic peritoneal lavage is traditionally the generally accepted standard for the diagnosis of possible abdominal injury, it has been replaced in most centers by CT. Diagnostic peritoneal lavage can yield false-negative results in injuries to retroperitoneal structures (e.g., kidneys, pancreas, duodenum) or the diaphragm. In addition, a positive peritoneal lavage occurs in up to 25% of patients with trivial injuries who do not require laparotomy, and may occur in patients with pelvic fractures or as a result of a traumatic peritoneal tap.

Postoperative Anastomotic Leaks

Common Causes

Complicated bariatric bypasses (weight reduction procedures)

Colonic resections for diverticulitis or rectal cancer

Colectomy for ulcerative colitis with creation of a J-pouch and ileo-anal anastomosis

Diverting colostomy/ileostomy (imaging required prior to closure to exclude a leak)

Esophagectomy

Gastrectomy

Heller myotomy

Approach to Diagnostic Imaging

■ 1. Digital fluoroscopy

- Multiple images can be obtained at various angles and degrees of magnification to show extravasation. Water-soluble contrast material must be used. Ionic contrast material is generally given, except to patients following esophagectomy and gastric pullup, in whom nonionic contrast is used because of the risk of aspiration. For the upper GI tract, the contrast material is administered by mouth; for colonic anastomoses, it is given by enema through a soft rubber-tipped catheter (generally a non-inflated Foley catheter).

- If the water-soluble examination is normal, thin barium is then administered

6

URINARY

N. Reed Dunnick

Dysuria

Common Causes

Urethritis (infection, catheters)
Cystitis (infection, radiation, chemicals, catheters, stones)
Prostatitis
Bladder tumor
Functional bladder syndrome

Approach to Diagnostic Imaging

 Caveat: In most cases, the cause of dysuria is evident from clinical examination and urinalysis, and no imaging procedures are necessary.

■ 1. Excretory urography or voiding cystourethrography

- Can demonstrate diffuse, irregular thickening of the bladder wall in inflammatory disease, as well as a lucent filling defect resulting from a bladder stone or tumor

Flank Pain

Common Causes

Trauma
Spontaneous renal hemorrhage
Obstructing ureteral calculus

Approach to Diagnostic Imaging

■ 1. Computed tomography

- Most sensitive single examination
- Unenhanced images to detect urolithiasis and hemorrhage
- Enhanced images often detect the etiology of spontaneous hemorrhage

■ 2. Ultrasound

- Relatively efficient for detecting renal masses or ureteral obstruction
- Useful when there is a need to avoid ionizing radiation, such as in examining pregnant women and children

 Caveat: Ultrasound is less sensitive than CT for the detection of renal masses.

Hematuria (Painless)

Common Causes

Neoplasm (kidney, ureter, bladder, urethra)
Glomerulonephritis
Vascular abnormality (aneurysm, malformation, arterial or venous occlusion)
Papillary necrosis
Urolithiasis

Approach to Diagnostic Imaging

■ 1. Computed tomography

- More sensitive than US for detecting renal masses
- If combined with an unenhanced examination, will also detect urinary tract calculi

■ 2. Ultrasound

- Relatively efficient imaging technique for detecting neoplastic renal masses and vascular anomalies

■ 3. Cystoscopy

- Required in any adult with unexplained hematuria because a normal US examination or cystogram does not exclude a bladder tumor or cystitis

Hematuria (Painful)

Common Causes

Ureteral calculus
Trauma
Infection (especially cystitis or urethritis)

Approach to Diagnostic Imaging

■ 1. Computed tomography (unenhanced)

- Can detect even poorly opaque stones (e.g., uric acid calculi)
- Can detect dilatation of the collecting system proximal to an obstructing stone
- Can detect secondary signs of ureteral obstruction such as perinephric stranding or extravasation
- Presence of tissue (edematous ureter) surrounding a calcification (rim sign) can differentiate a ureteral calculus from a phlebolith or other extraurinary calcification
- Stones larger than 5 mm may require endoscopic removal
- Can detect extraurinary cause of abdominal pain such as cholelithiasis and appendicitis
- May be used in patients in whom intravascular contrast material is contraindicated

■ 2. Ultrasound

- Can demonstrate the presence and degree of ureteral dilatation proximal to an impacted stone
- Can demonstrate a stone as an echogenic focus with acoustic shadowing in the patient with a nonopaque, completely obstructing stone causing loss of ipsilateral kidney function
- Transvaginal US may be used to increase the sensitivity for detection of distal ureteral stones
- Ureteral stones may be obscured by bowel gas
- US may be the procedure of choice for pregnant patients

Renal Failure (Acute)

Presenting Signs and Symptoms

Rapid, steadily increasing azotemia, with or without oliguria

Common Causes

PRERENAL

Hypovolemia (diarrhea, vomiting, hemorrhage, over-diuresis, pancreatitis, peritonitis)

Vasodilatation (sepsis, drugs, anaphylaxis)

Cardiac (congestive heart failure, myocardial infarction, cardiac tamponade)

Renal hypoperfusion (renal artery obstruction)

RENAL

Acute tubular injury (ischemia, toxins, hemoglobinuria, myoglobinuria, radiocontrast agents)

Acute glomerulonephritis

Acute tubular nephritis (drug reaction, pyelonephritis, papillary necrosis)

Precipitation of substances within the kidney (calcium, urates, myeloma protein)

Arterial or venous obstruction

Disseminated intravascular coagulopathy with cortical necrosis

POSTRENAL

Calculi

Prostatism

Neoplasm (bladder, pelvic, retroperitoneal)

Retroperitoneal fibrosis

Urethral or bladder neck obstruction

Approach to Diagnostic Imaging

■ 1. Ultrasound

- Imaging procedure of choice for assessing renal size, identifying renal parenchymal disease (diffuse increase in echogenicity with loss of corticomedullary differentiation), and excluding hydronephrosis (postrenal cause)

> **Note:** In patients with acute renal failure and *large* (>12cm) or normal-sized kidneys, biopsy is often required for definitive diagnosis of renal parenchymal disease; patients with *small* (<9cm) kidneys usually have irreversible end-stage renal disease and do not benefit from biopsy.

- If a vascular cause is suggested clinically, color Doppler studies may demonstrate patency or occlusion of the renal artery or vein. If this is unsuccessful, radionuclide renal scan or magnetic resonance imaging can show these vessels.

 Caveat: Although arteriography and venography are more definitive tests for vascular occlusion, some physicians prefer not to use radiographic contrast agents in patients with acute renal failure.

Renal Failure (Chronic)

Presenting Signs and Symptoms

Irreversible loss of renal function (uremia)
Neuromuscular (peripheral neuropathy, muscle cramps,
   convulsions, encephalopathy)
Gastrointestinal (anorexia, nausea and vomiting, peptic
   ulcer, unpleasant taste in the mouth)
Cardiopulmonary (congestive heart failure, hypertension,
   pericarditis, pleural effusion)
Skin (uremic frost, pruritus)
Secondary hyperparathyroidism

Common Causes

Diabetic nephropathy
Hypertension
Glomerulonephritis
Polycystic kidney disease (autosomal dominant)

Approach to Diagnostic Imaging

■ 1. Ultrasound

- ■ Imaging procedure of choice for assessing kidney size (usually small kidneys in chronic
  renal failure), as well as detecting hydronephrosis secondary to obstruction (especially
  in patients with risk factors such as known or
  suspected pelvic malignancy, or bladder outlet
  obstruction)

Incontinence

Common Causes

WOMEN

Pelvic relaxation (childbearing)
Urethral diverticulum
Urethritis/cystitis

MEN

Following prostatectomy or repair of urethral stricture

BOTH

Neurogenic bladder
Medications (e.g., antipsychotics, diuretics)

Approach to Diagnostic Imaging

■ 1. Voiding cystourethrography

- Confirms the presence of incontinence
- Can be used to classify the type of incontinence and identify the phase during which it occurs (filling, straining, coughing)
- Assesses the size, contour, capacity, and contractility of the bladder

■ 2. Ultrasound

- Not used as primary imaging technique because it cannot directly visualize urine loss or identify the phase during which incontinence occurs
- Can detect urethral diverticula and determine bladder wall thickness
- Better for evaluating dilatation of the more proximal urinary tract and possible renal parenchymal loss

Note: Some urologists prefer performing urodynamic studies instead of, or in addition to, imaging procedures.

Pyelonephritis (Acute)

Presenting Signs and Symptoms

Rapid onset of fever and chills, flank pain, nausea and
vomiting

Pyuria with white blood cell casts

Common Causes

Ascending urinary tract infection (especially *Escherichia
coli*)

Obstruction is a predisposing factor (strictures, calculi,
neurogenic bladder, vesicoureteral reflux)

Approach to Diagnostic Imaging

 Caveat: Uncomplicated infection requires *no*
imaging; imaging studies are indicated *only* in
patients who fail to respond to treatment or who
are severely ill.

■ 1. Computed tomography

- ■ May demonstrate a complicating renal or perirenal
  abscess as a thick-walled fluid collection within
  the kidney that may extend to the perirenal space

Note: The "pre-abscess" state of focal bacterial infection appears as a focal wedge-shaped or rounded area of decreased density. Uncomplicated disease appears as swollen, edematous kidneys, usually with patchy areas of decreased density or a striated parenchymal nephrogram.

■ 2. Ultrasound

- Also can demonstrate renal or perirenal abscess (but less sensitive than CT for detecting subtle changes in the renal parenchyma associated with uncomplicated pyelonephritis)
- Can efficiently diagnose hydronephrosis if it is unclear whether urinary tract obstruction is a predisposing factor to the development of infection

Pyelonephritis (Chronic)

Presenting Signs and Symptoms

Progressive renal failure

History of recurrent urinary tract infections (infrequently obtained except in children with vesicoureteral reflux)

Pyuria with white blood cell casts

Common Causes

Recurrent urinary tract infections (especially when associated with obstructive uropathy)

Vesicoureteral reflux in children

Approach to Diagnostic Imaging

■ 1. Computed tomography

- Demonstrates small and atrophic kidney on the affected side. Focal coarse renal scarring with clubbing of the underlying calyx is characteristic

> **Note:** Although chronic pyelonephritis is typically lobar, with normal lobes interposed between diseased ones, there may be generalized calyceal dilatation with an irregular renal margin.

■ 2. Ultrasound

- Alternative approach that shows focal loss of renal parenchyma, increased echogenicity in the area of the scar, and extension of the central renal sinus echoes to the periphery of the kidney in the area of abnormality

Pyonephrosis

Presenting Sign and Symptom

Signs of infection in an obstructed kidney

Approach to Diagnostic Imaging

■ 1. Ultrasound

- Preferred initial imaging modality for demonstrating the pathognomonic appearance of a dilated collecting system with layering of echogenic pus and debris

■ 2. Computed tomography

- May be superior to US in determining the precise site and cause of an obstruction and in defining an extrarenal abscess or fluid collection

■ 3. Interventional procedure

- Placement of a ureteral stent or percutaneous nephrostomy catheter to relieve the obstruction (combined with antibiotic therapy) should be performed *promptly* to prevent rapid destruction of the renal parenchyma that can result if the condition is not properly treated

Renal Abscess

Presenting Signs and Symptoms

Fever, leukocytosis, and flank pain

Frequently, a history of prior antibiotic therapy with relapse on cessation

Approach to Diagnostic Imaging

■ 1. Computed tomography

- Preferred study for demonstrating the thick-walled, low-attenuation mass within the kidney that may extend to the perirenal space (usually thickening of Gerota's fascia and strands of increased density in the adjacent fat)

- Gas within the mass is virtually pathognomonic of renal abscess

 Caveat: There is *no* indication for excretory urography in the patient with a suspected renal abscess.

■ 2. Ultrasound

- Alternative method for demonstrating a renal or perinephric abscess, but less sensitive than CT

■ 3. Interventional radiology

- Percutaneous drainage using CT or US guidance is the preferred method of therapy because it provides satisfactory clinical results using local anesthesia and precludes the need for open surgical drainage

Perinephric (Perirenal) Abscess

Presenting Signs and Symptoms

Fever, leukocytosis and flank pain (at least a 2-week history of symptoms of urinary tract infection)

Frequently a history of prior antibiotic therapy with relapse on cessation

Referred pain to the thorax, groin, thigh, or hip (indicating that the disease has spread beyond the confines of the kidney)

Common Causes

PRIMARY

Forms when an intrarenal abscess breaks through the renal capsule into the perirenal space

SECONDARY

Hematogenous spread to the perirenal space from a distant focus or direct extension from an infection in an adjacent organ (e.g., ruptured appendix or diverticulitis)

Predisposing Factors

Staghorn calculus
Diabetes mellitus
Pyonephrosis
Neurogenic bladder
Immunocompromised patient

Approach to Diagnostic Imaging

■ **1. Computed tomography**

- Preferred study for demonstrating the low-attenuation mass (usually with an enhancing wall) as well as precisely defining the boundaries of the inflammatory process by detecting any extension into the psoas muscle and true pelvis
- Gas within the mass is virtually pathognomonic of renal abscess

■ **2. Interventional radiology**

- Percutaneous drainage using CT or US guidance is the preferred method of therapy because it provides satisfactory clinical results using local anesthesia, and precludes the need for open surgical drainage

Urinary Tract Infection (Infant)

Major Predisposing Factors

Obstruction of urinary tract (structural or functional)
Vesicoureteral reflux

Approach to Diagnostic Imaging

■ 1. Radionuclide or voiding cystography

- Demonstrates the presence and degree of any observed vesicoureteral reflux

Note: Radionuclide cystography is the most sensitive imaging technique for showing vesicoureteral reflux and delivers a substantially lower radiation dose to the gonads. It is especially valuable when multiple follow-up studies are needed to evaluate progression of disease and response to therapy.

■ 2. Ultrasound

- Preferred imaging study for detecting underlying anatomic abnormalities and significant renal scarring (simple, noninvasive, no ionizing radiation)

Note: A complete investigation of the urinary tract is important after an episode of urinary tract infection in an infant because of the relatively high probability of an underlying anatomic abnormality.

Urinary Tract Infection (Female Child)

Approach to Diagnostic Imaging

Caveat: There is controversy as to whether female children (who constitute the overwhelming majority of those affected) should be subjected to radiographic imaging after an initial urinary tract infection (because at least 75% have no abnormality and the risk of developing reflux nephropathy in girls with normal urinary tracts at the time of their first urinary tract infection is very small). *But* it is generally agreed that a workup of the urinary tract *is* indicated for repeat or relapsing infections.

■ 1. Radionuclide or voiding cystography

- Demonstrates the presence and degree of any observed vesicoureteral reflux

> **Note:** Radionuclide cystography is the most sensitive imaging technique for showing vesicoureteral reflux and delivers a substantially lower radiation dose to the gonads. It is especially valuable when multiple follow-up studies are needed to evaluate progression of disease and response to therapy.

■ 2. Ultrasound

- Preferred imaging study for detecting underlying anatomic abnormalities and significant renal scarring (simple, noninvasive, no ionizing radiation)

Urinary Tract Infection (Male Child)

Major Predisposing Factors

Obstruction of urinary tract (structural or functional)
Vesicoureteral reflux

Approach to Diagnostic Imaging

■ 1. Radionuclide or voiding cystography

- Demonstrates the presence and degree of any observed vesicoureteral reflux

Note: Radionuclide cystography is the most sensitive imaging technique for showing vesicoureteral reflux and delivers a substantially lower radiation dose to the gonads. It is especially valuable when multiple follow-up studies are needed to evaluate progression of disease and response to therapy.

■ 2. Ultrasound

- Preferred imaging study for detecting underlying anatomic abnormalities/significant renal scarring (simple, noninvasive, no ionizing radiation)

Urinary Tract Infection (Older Child/Teenager)

Approach to Diagnostic Imaging

■ 1. Ultrasound

- A normal study indicates that there is no reflux nephropathy and that the child (by this age) is at little risk of developing intrinsic renal disease in the future

---

Note: This is the only study needed if the child has only lower urinary tract signs and symptoms.

Upper Urinary Tract Infection (Adult)

Presenting Signs and Symptoms

Fever
Flank pain
Pyuria

Indications for Imaging

Infection requiring hospitalization
Impaired renal function
Relapsing infection
Infection in a male

 Caveat: Uncomplicated infection in a woman requires *no* imaging (and often shows no abnormalities).

Approach to Diagnostic Imaging

■ 1. Excretory urography

- Provides information on structure and function of urinary tract
- Normal examination in a patient with acute urinary tract infection excludes pyonephrosis and other severe renal infections (although it does not eliminate the possibility of vesicoureteral reflux or a perinephric inflammatory process)

■ 2. Ultrasound

- Preferred imaging modality for evaluating the critically ill patient with suspected upper urinary tract infection
- Preferred imaging modality for evaluating patients with impaired renal function
- May demonstrate even minimal dilatation of the intrarenal collecting system, renal stones, and intrarenal masses
- Excellent method for delineating and guiding drainage of a perinephric abscess

■ 3. Computed tomography

- Indicated if US or excretory urography is normal yet there is strong clinical suspicion of an infectious process involving the kidney or the perinephric space
- Excellent method for delineating and guiding drainage of a perinephric abscess

Renal Mass

Presenting Signs and Symptoms

Flank pain
Hematuria
Palpable mass
Fever (suggests renal abscess)
Often discovered incidentally in an asymptomatic patient by US, or CT performed for unrelated abdominal pathology

Common Causes

Cyst
Neoplasm (benign or malignant)
Abscess

Major Imaging Goal

To separate benign renal cysts (the large majority of renal masses) from solid or cystic neoplasms

> **Note:** The unequivocal imaging diagnosis of a benign cyst usually precludes the need for surgical confirmation.

Approach to Diagnostic Imaging

■ 1. Ultrasound

- Highly accurate for demonstrating the characteristic findings of a simple cyst:
  - Absence of internal echoes
  - Strong, sharply defined distal wall with smooth, distinct margins
  - Enhanced through-transmission of the sound beam
  - Posterior acoustic enhancement
  - Spherical or slightly ovoid shape

 Caveats: (1) Hemorrhagic or infected cysts may be indistinguishable sonographically from solid benign and malignant neoplasms and inflammatory masses; (2) US may be inadequate in obese patients.

■ 2. Computed tomography

- More sensitive than US for detecting renal masses
- Highly accurate for demonstrating the characteristic findings of a simple cyst as a nonenhancing mass of water attenuation with clearly defined margins, compared with an enhancing mass that is typical of a solid neoplasm

Note: Although generally considered the "gold standard" for evaluating renal mass lesions, CT is more expensive than screening US and requires intravenous contrast material. Therefore, in many centers, CT is indicated only when the US examination is indeterminate or technically inadequate due to obesity or overlying gas. Because CT is more sensitive than US for detecting a renal mass, it may be used in patients with a negative US examination for whom there is a strong clinical suspicion of a renal mass.

Renal Cyst

Presenting Signs and Symptoms

Asymptomatic (discovered incidentally during US or CT performed for unrelated abdominal pathology)

Occasionally, a palpable mass, flank discomfort or pain, or hematuria

Common Causes

Unknown

Approach to Diagnostic Imaging

Note: The imaging goal is to separate benign renal cysts (the large majority of renal masses) from malignant neoplasms, because the unequivocal imaging diagnosis of a benign cyst usually precludes the need for surgical confirmation.

Approach to Diagnostic Imaging

■ **1. Ultrasound**

- Highly accurate for demonstrating the characteristic findings of a simple cyst:
    - Absence of internal echoes
    - Strong, sharply defined distal wall with smooth, distinct margins
    - Enhanced through-transmission of the sound beam
    - Posterior acoustic enhancement
    - Spherical or slightly ovoid shape

 Caveat: Hemorrhagic or infected cysts may be indistinguishable sonographically from solid benign and malignant neoplasms and inflammatory masses.

■ 2. Computed tomography

- Indicated if the US appearance is atypical for a simple cyst (thick wall, calcification, internal debris)
- Demonstrates a hemorrhagic cyst as a homogeneous mass that appears hyperdense to normal renal parenchyma on unenhanced scans and hypodense on contrast studies
- Gas within a thick-walled mass strongly suggests an infected cyst

Cancer of the Kidney

Presenting Signs and Symptoms

Hematuria

Flank pain

Palpable mass

Fever of unknown origin

Increasingly being detected incidentally in asymptomatic patients during US or CT performed for unrelated abdominal pathology

Approach to Diagnostic Imaging

■ 1. Computed tomography

- Contrast-enhanced CT is more sensitive than US for detecting renal masses
- When combined with an unenhanced examination, CT can distinguish hemorrhagic cysts from solid tumors

■ 2. Ultrasound

- Can demonstrate a tumor as a solid, heterogeneous, hypoechoic or mildly hyperechoic mass that may contain cystic areas representing hemorrhage or necrosis

■ 3. Magnetic resonance imaging

- As sensitive as CT for detecting renal masses
- Useful for patients with a contraindication to iodinated intravascular contrast material

Staging

■ 1. Computed tomography or magnetic resonance imaging

- Most effective staging procedures for demonstrating the presence and extent of extrarenal spread of tumor (including invasion of the renal vein and inferior vena cava, which is still a surgically curable stage of disease if there are no distant metastases)

Note: Doppler US also can detect echogenic tumor thrombus within venous structures.

- MRI may prove to be accurate in determining whether the small opacities seen in the perinephric space on CT in many patients represent patent vessels or lymphadenopathy
- Chest CT should be performed for detection of pulmonary metastases prior to any potentially curative surgical procedure

■ 2. Radionuclide bone scan

- Should be performed to detect any skeletal metastases prior to any potentially curative surgical procedure

■ 3. Arteriography

- Presurgical embolization of a tumor may dramatically reduce its vascularity, making resection easier by diminishing blood loss

Medullary Cystic Disease

Presenting Signs and Symptoms

Polyuria (with urinary sodium wasting)
Unexplained uremia
Retarded growth and evidence of bone disease
Symptoms usually begin before age 20

Common Causes

Genetic or congenital

Approach to Diagnostic Imaging

■ 1. Ultrasound

- May demonstrate the multiple medullary cysts within small, smooth kidneys or merely generalized increased echogenicity of the renal parenchyma (representing diffuse atrophy)

Note: Because the cysts may be few and small, they often cannot be detected by US.

Multicystic Dysplastic Kidney

Presenting Signs and Symptoms

Palpable abdominal mass in a neonate (asymptomatic)
Usually unilateral (can be bilateral or segmental)

Common Causes

Congenital developmental defect (resulting from occlusion of the fetal ureter, usually before 8–10 weeks of gestation)

Approach to Diagnostic Imaging

■ **1. Ultrasound**

- Demonstrates numerous cysts of various sizes with variable amounts of intervening dysplastic renal tissue

Polycystic Kidney Disease (Adult)

Presenting Signs and Symptoms

Initially asymptomatic (may be discovered incidentally on abdominal US or CT performed for another reason)

Onset in early or middle life with symptoms related to the effects of the cysts (lumbar discomfort or pain, hematuria, infection, or colic due to nephrolithiasis)

Hypertension (50% at time of diagnosis)

Progressive renal dysfunction with uremic symptoms

Cysts may also be present in the liver (in 50%)

Aneurysms of the circle of Willis (in 15%) that may rupture to produce subarachnoid hemorrhage

Common Cause

Autosomal dominant

Approach to Diagnostic Imaging

■ 1. Ultrasound or computed tomography

- Demonstrates progressive replacement of the renal parenchyma by multiple noncommunicating cysts of various sizes that commonly contain internal hemorrhage
- Can detect associated cysts in the liver

Polycystic Kidney Disease (Childhood)

Presenting Signs and Symptoms

In *neonates,* there is renal dysfunction with pulmonary hypoplasia (often a protuberant abdomen with huge kidneys and an enlarged liver)

In *children,* signs and symptoms of portal hypertension (due to progressive hepatic fibrosis) become more prominent and renal insufficiency is only mild or moderate

Common Cause

Autosomal recessive

Approach to Diagnostic Imaging

■ 1. Ultrasound

- *Prenatal* studies in late pregnancy usually can permit a presumptive diagnosis
- In young children, ultrasound shows characteristic bilaterally enlarged, echogenic kidneys with dilated renal tubules arranged in a radiating pattern (may be so dilated as to appear as individual structures)
- In older children and adolescents, ultrasound can show cysts in the kidneys and liver, as well as secondary signs, associated with hepatic fibrosis and portal hypertension

---

Note: A final diagnosis may require renal and liver biopsies.

Atheroembolic Renal Disease

Presenting Signs and Symptoms

Sudden or gradual development of progressive renal failure (depending on amount of atheromatous material obstructing the renal arteries)

May show evidence of embolic disease elsewhere (cholesterol emboli visible on fundoscopic examination, neurologic deficits, toe gangrene, livedo reticularis)

Usually hypertension

Common Causes

Spontaneous embolization of atheromatous plaques

Embolization subsequent to vascular surgery, angioplasty, or arteriography

Approach to Diagnostic Imaging

■ 1. Computed tomography

- Demonstrates a resulting renal infarction as a wedge-shaped area of low attenuation within an otherwise normal kidney

> **Note:** Typically, the outer 2–4 mm of cortex are preserved, even if the entire renal artery is occluded, because capsular branches remain patent and enhance the outer rim of the kidney.

■ 2. Arteriography

- Defines vascular occlusion
- Thrombolytic therapy is less likely to be successful with embolic disease than with acute thrombosis

Nephrosclerosis (Malignant)

Presenting Signs and Symptoms

Severe hypertension and rapidly progressive renal failure

Common Causes

Accelerated cardiovascular disease in the course of primary
hypertension (especially untreated)

May arise from secondary hypertension (due to acute
glomerulonephritis, chronic renal failure, renovascular
hypertension, vasculitis)

Approach to Diagnostic Imaging

 Caveat: Imaging is seldom of value.

■ 1. Arteriography

- Demonstrates increased tortuosity and more rapid
  tapering of intrarenal arteries
- May show filling defects and loss of cortical vessels

Renal Cortical Necrosis

Presenting Signs and Symptoms

Abrupt anuria with gross hematuria and flank pain

Common Causes

NEONATES

Abruptio placentae
Bacterial sepsis

CHILDREN

Infections
Extracellular volume depletion
Shock
Hemolytic-uremic syndrome

ADULTS

Accidents of pregnancy (abruptio placentae, placenta previa, uterine hemorrhage, puerperal sepsis, amniotic fluid embolism, intrauterine death, preeclampsia)
Bacterial sepsis
Hemolytic-uremic syndrome
Hyperacute transplant rejection
Burns
Pancreatitis
Poisoning (phosphorus, arsenic)

Approach to Diagnostic Imaging

■ 1. Ultrasound

- Initially shows enlarged kidneys (renal size progressively diminishes and may be reduced to about 50% of normal by 6–8 weeks)

■ 2. Plain abdominal radiograph

- Demonstrates characteristic late (6–8 weeks) sign of calcification that is often linear and is most marked at the corticomedullary junction

Renal Infarction

Presenting Signs and Symptoms

Steady aching flank pain localized to affected renal area

May be asymptomatic (if a small branch of the renal artery is occluded)

Usually, fever, nausea and vomiting, leukocytosis, proteinuria, and microscopic hematuria

Common Causes

Renal artery occlusion (embolic, thrombotic, arteritis, sickle cell disease)

Iatrogenic (after surgery, angioplasty, selective arteriography)

Approach to Diagnostic Imaging

■ 1. Computed tomography

- Demonstrates an infarction as a wedge-shaped area of low attenuation within an otherwise normal kidney

Note: Typically, the outer 2–4 mm of cortex are preserved, even if the entire renal artery is occluded, because capsular branches remain patent and enhance the outer rim of the kidney.

■ 2. Arteriography

- Defines vascular occlusion and often allows a diagnosis of vasculitis or emboli
- May be useful for thrombolytic therapy if the infarction is due to acute thrombosis

 Caveat: There is *no* indication for excretory urography because there is no renal function in the face of occlusion of the main renal artery.

Renal Vein Thrombosis

Presenting Signs and Symptoms
ACUTE (ANY AGE)

Flank pain
Fever
Hematuria, oliguria
Edema
Leukocytosis
Renal failure

SLOWLY PROGRESSIVE (ADULTS)

Gradual onset of proteinuria
Deteriorating glomerular filtration rate
Nephrotic syndrome

Common Causes
CHILDREN

Diarrhea, dehydration
Hypercoagulability

ADULTS

Membranous glomerulonephritis
Pregnancy
Oral contraceptive use
Trauma
Extrinsic compression (lymph nodes, aortic aneurysm,
    tumor)
Invasion by renal cell carcinoma

Approach to Diagnostic Imaging

■ 1. Ultrasound

- Demonstrates an enlarged kidney in acute disease and an atrophic kidney in slowly progressive disease

---

Note: If venous collateral vessels provide adequate drainage, the kidney may be unaffected.

- Doppler studies may permit the direct detection of clot within the renal veins

■ 2. Computed tomography

- Absence of opacification of the renal vein on contrast-enhanced study

■ 3. Magnetic resonance imaging

- Detection of an abnormally strong signal from the renal veins (normally a dark flow void), suggesting stasis of flow
- Slow-flowing laminar blood (paradoxical brightness) may outline a lower-signal clot within it

■ 4. Venography

- May demonstrate thrombus within the renal vein, or absence of venous opacification implying obstruction

Renovascular Hypertension

Clinical Indications Suggestive of a Renovascular Cause

Onset of hypertension in a previously normotensive person older than age 50

Onset of hypertension in a person younger than age 30

Women between ages 30 and 50 who have no family history of hypertension (fibromuscular hyperplasia)

Rapid acceleration or severe hypertension

Presence of an abdominal or flank bruit

Deteriorating renal function

Poor control of blood pressure with medical therapy

Severe hypertensive retinopathy

Common Causes

Renal artery stenosis

Fibromuscular dysplasia

Takayasu's aortitis

Approach to Diagnostic Imaging

> **Note:** Many radiographic screening tests have been used in patients with suspected renovascular hypertension; there is no consensus as to which is best. Choice may reflect local institutional bias, available equipment, physician interest or expertise, and characteristics of the patient population.

■ **1. Radionuclide renogram with captopril**

- Noninvasive screening test

■ **2. Doppler ultrasound**

- Limited by operator dependence

■ 3. Arteriography

- "Gold standard" for detecting renal artery stenosis (the presence of renal artery stenosis in a hypertensive patient does not necessarily mean that the patient has renovascular hypertension)

Note: Arteriography is infrequently used as a screening procedure because of its highly invasive nature.

■ 4. Computed tomography angiography

- Noninvasive technique that can detect renal artery stenosis, including fibromuscular dysplasia

■ 5. Magnetic resonance angiography

- Noninvasive technique that can detect renal artery stenosis
- Resolution insufficient to detect rare segmental stenoses in renal artery branch vessels
- Does not require iodinated intravascular contrast material and is safer for use in azotemic patients

■ 6. Interventional radiology

- Percutaneous renal angioplasty has become a widespread technique for the nonsurgical therapy of renal artery stenosis. The overall technical success rate is reported to be 80–95%, with 10–20% of stenoses recurring (most often when there has been incomplete dilatation of the lesion). Major complications occur in about 5% of patients.

Bladder Trauma

Presenting Signs and Symptoms

Gross hematuria
Lower abdominal or suprapubic pain
Hypotension
Pelvic fracture

Approach to Diagnostic Imaging

■ 1. Cystography

- Sensitive imaging procedure for detecting extravasation of contrast material indicating intraperitoneal or extraperitoneal (more common) rupture

 Caveat: The urethra should *never* be catheterized if a urethral injury is suspected. Under such circumstances, the proper approach is to perform retrograde urethrography. Only if the urethra is shown to be normal should a catheter be passed into the bladder.

■ 2. Computed tomography

- In addition to demonstrating extravasation of contrast material, CT can precisely define the site and extent of extraperitoneal perivesical hematoma

Note: CT of the abdomen and pelvis is usually performed to evaluate injury to other organs after major abdominal trauma.

Caveat: Bladder rupture may be missed on CT (or cystography) if the bladder is decompressed by a catheter or if it is incompletely filled. With current-generation CT scanners, the entire abdomen and pelvis may be imaged before contrast material reaches the bladder. Therefore, filling the bladder with dilute contrast through a Foley catheter or taking delayed images may be required to evaluate the bladder.

■ 3. Arteriography

- Indicated in the patient with a significant pelvic hematoma who has a decreasing hematocrit and no other apparent source of blood loss
- Therapeutic embolization of a bleeding vessel may preclude the need for surgery

Renal Trauma (Blunt)

Presenting Signs and Symptoms

Hematuria

Flank pain and tenderness

Hypotension or shock

Associated injuries (skeletal fracture, signs of injury to the spleen, liver, or gastrointestinal tract)

Approach to Diagnostic Imaging

GENERAL APPROACH

1. *Unstable* patients should have immediate surgical exploration without waiting for imaging studies

2. In stable patients with *microscopic* hematuria and no suspected associated injuries or fractures, radiographic contrast studies have a very *low* likelihood of detecting significant renal injury

3. In stable patients with *gross* hematuria or microscopic hematuria and shock, the yield of radiographic contrast studies is sufficiently *high* to influence further therapy

■ 1. Computed tomography

■ Most versatile imaging technique that, in addition to demonstrating morphologic and functional abnormalities of the kidneys, can show intraperitoneal and extraperitoneal hemorrhage, free intraperitoneal gas, and injuries to the liver, spleen, pancreas, and gastrointestinal tract

Note: Unsuspected injuries to other organs are common and are more likely to be revealed by CT than any other imaging modality.

■ 2. Arteriography

- Seldom needed as a diagnostic test, since the integrity of the renal artery can be predicted on the basis of the CT examination
- May be indicated as a prelude to surgery in a patient with a nonfunctioning kidney presumed to be due to vascular occlusion

 Caveat: In 90% of patients with complete arterial occlusion, renal function is irreversibly lost after 2 h of ischemia. Therefore, the need for immediate surgery must be balanced against the time required to complete an arteriographic examination.

- Embolization of a bleeding vessel may permit stabilization of the patient and preclude the need for surgery

Note: In patients in whom iodinated contrast material is contraindicated, US may be performed to evaluate renal morphology, and radionuclide scanning may be employed to assess renal perfusion and function.

Renal Trauma (Penetrating)

Presenting Signs and Symptoms

Hematuria
Flank pain and tenderness
Hypotension or shock

Approach to Diagnostic Imaging

Caveat: In up to 6% of patients, significant occult injuries to the kidney are not suggested on clinical inspection of the wound. The absence of hematuria does *not* exclude renal injury. Studies have shown that (1) 30% of patients with penetrating flank and back trauma without hematuria had renal pedicle injuries; and (2) 15–42% of patients with flank or back trauma manifest only microscopic hematuria.

■ 1. Computed tomography

- Contrast-enhanced scans are the imaging procedure of choice for demonstrating renal laceration and extravasation of contrast material from the pelvicalyceal system

■ 2. Arteriography

- Needed to demonstrate a bleeding vessel
- Therapeutic embolization of an actively bleeding vessel may preclude the need for surgery

Urethral Trauma

Presenting Signs and Symptoms

Inability to urinate
Blood at the urethral meatus
Elevation of the prostate on digital rectal examination
Perineal swelling or hematoma
Pelvic fracture

Approach to Diagnostic Imaging

■ 1. Retrograde urethrography

- Imaging procedure of choice for demonstrating extravasation of contrast material through a partial or complete urethral tear

 Caveat: If urethral injury is suspected, a retrograde urethrogram should always be obtained prior to transurethral bladder catheterization. If the bladder of a patient with a urethral injury is full, suprapubic catheterization may be performed.

Glomerulonephritis (Acute)

Presenting Signs and Symptoms

Sudden onset of hematuria (dark urine with red cell casts), oliguria

Edema

Hypertension

Elevated blood urea nitrogen and creatinine

Common Causes

Prior beta-hemolytic streptococcal infection

Other prior infection (bacterial, viral, parasitic)

Multisystem disease (systemic lupus erythematosus, vasculitis, Henoch-Schönlein purpura, Goodpasture's syndrome)

Approach to Diagnostic Imaging

■ 1. Ultrasound

■ May aid in distinguishing acute disease (usually normal or slightly enlarged kidneys) from an exacerbation of chronic disease (small kidneys)

Glomerulonephritis (Chronic)

Presenting Signs and Symptoms

Insidious onset of slowly progressive impairment of renal failure associated with peripheral edema

May be discovered incidentally on urinalysis in an asymptomatic patient (proteinuria, possibly hematuria)

Common Cause

Most frequently, develops weeks or months after an episode of acute glomerulonephritis

Approach to Diagnostic Imaging

■ 1. Ultrasound

- Demonstrates the nonspecific pattern of bilateral small kidneys (as with other causes of chronic renal failure)

Note: US can exclude obstructive hydronephrosis as the underlying cause of progressive renal failure.

Hydronephrosis

Presenting Signs and Symptoms

ACUTE

Colicky pain

CHRONIC

Asymptomatic

Recurrent attacks of dull flank pain (resulting stasis may lead to formation of calculi and secondary infection)

Common Causes

NONOBSTRUCTIVE

Vesicoureteral reflux

Primary megacalyces

OBSTRUCTIVE

Obstruction at the ureteropelvic junction (fibrous band, aberrant vessel, ureteral kinking, renal pelvis stone or tumor)

Distal obstruction (stone, tumor, benign prostatic hyperplasia, ureteral stricture, retroperitoneal fibrosis, bladder outlet obstruction); in pregnancy, transient involvement of right ureter

Approach to Diagnostic Imaging

■ 1. Ultrasound

- Preferred initial imaging modality for detecting urinary tract dilatation
- Dilatation of the renal pelvis appears as separation of the normal sinus echogenicity by anechoic urine in the collecting system

■ 2. Computed tomography

- Frequently permits identification of the cause of the obstruction, in addition to demonstrating dilatation of the ureter and collecting system

Medullary Sponge Kidney

Presenting Signs and Symptoms

Usually asymptomatic

Nephrocalcinosis may lead to symptomatic complications such as colic, hematuria, and infection (from urinary stasis)

Common Cause

Congenital dysplastic dilatation of the collecting tubules

Approach to Diagnostic Imaging

■ 1. Computed tomography

- Shows characteristic striations or saccular papillary collections of contrast material (most commonly bilateral and symmetric)
- Preliminary (scout) radiograph may show calcifications in the dilated tubules in the medullary pyramids

Note: US is seldom useful because the cysts are small and located deep in the medulla; it may show papillary stones as echogenic foci.

Nephrocalcinosis

Presenting Signs and Symptoms

Asymptomatic (unless complicated by hematuria, obstruction, or infection)

Common Causes

Pathologic deposition of calcium may occur in
Medulla
Hyperparathyroidism
Medullary sponge kidney
Renal tubular acidosis
Milk-alkali syndrome
Hypervitaminosis D
Hypercalcemic/hypercalciuric states
Pyramids
Hyperuricemia
Infection (tuberculosis)
Sickle cell disease
Cortex
Acute cortical necrosis
Chronic glomerulonephritis

Approach to Diagnostic Imaging

■ 1. Plain abdominal radiograph, ultrasound, or computed tomography

- Plain abdominal radiographs are the least expensive and most readily available, but US and especially CT are more sensitive for detecting subtle calcification in the renal parenchyma
- Calculi appear opaque on plain radiographs, as echogenic lesions with acoustic shadowing on US, and as high-attenuation lesions on CT

Nephrolithiasis
(Urinary Calculi)

Presenting Signs and Symptoms

Asymptomatic (if not causing obstruction or passing down the ureter)

Renal colic (excruciating intermittent pain, usually originating in the flank or kidney area and radiating to the groin)

Hematuria

Chills and fever

Nausea, vomiting, and abdominal distension (clinical picture of adynamic ileus)

Common Types

Calcium oxalate or calcium phosphate (80%)

Struvite (magnesium ammonium phosphate) (13%)

Uric acid (5%)

Cystine (2%)

Approach to Diagnostic Imaging

■ 1. Computed tomography (unenhanced)

- Most sensitive method for detecting urinary tract calculi (even "radiolucent" stones are readily visible on CT)
- Can detect dilatation of the collecting system or ureter proximal to an obstructing stone
- Can detect rupture of the collecting system
- Can detect extraurinary causes of abdominal pain
- No risk of reaction to iodinated contrast material

■ 2. Ultrasound

- Demonstrates both opaque and lucent stones as echodensities with acoustic shadowing
- Shows the degree of ureteral dilatation proximal to an obstruction

 Caveat: US may fail to detect small stones in the renal pelvis that do not cast acoustic shadows and thus blend in with renal sinus fat.

Retroperitoneal Hemorrhage

Presenting Signs and Symptoms

Abdominal or back pain, often with symptoms of hypotension

Common Causes

Rupture of abdominal aortic aneurysm
Trauma
Coagulopathy (anticoagulant medication or intrinsic blood dyscrasia)
Hemorrhage into renal or retroperitoneal neoplasm
Pancreatitis
Iatrogenic (following groin puncture for arteriography or cardiac catheterization, a hematoma can spread from the pelvis into any of the retroperitoneal compartments)

Approach to Diagnostic Imaging

■ 1. Computed tomography

- Procedure of choice for demonstrating a ruptured aortic aneurysm, as well as for identifying most other morphologic causes of retroperitoneal hemorrhage
- Clearly shows the location, size, and extent of the hematoma

■ 2. Ultrasound

- Best technique for evaluating the groin after femoral vein puncture
- Procedure of choice for detecting arteriovenous fistulas and pseudoaneurysms
- Of limited use in the retroperitoneum in obese patients
- May be difficult to differentiate a hematoma from other retroperitoneal masses (tumor, abscess)

■ 3. Arteriography

- Indicated if CT suggests a discrete source of bleeding that could be treated with embolization (pseudoaneurysm, hemorrhage arising from a neoplasm)

■ 4. Magnetic resonance angiography

- May be an alternative for imaging major vessels noninvasively

 Caveat: Unstable patients with massive hemorrhage should have emergency surgery without any diagnostic imaging studies.

Tubulointerstitial Nephritis (Acute Tubular Necrosis)

Presenting Signs and Symptoms

Reversible renal failure, with or without oliguria

Symptoms vary with underlying cause (e.g., fever, rash, and arthralgia if cause is an allergic reaction to a drug)

Common Causes

Drug-induced (amphotericin, aminoglycosides, penicillins, sulfonamides, diuretics, nonsteroidal antiinflammatory drugs, heavy metals, radiocontrast agents)

Systemic infections

Pyelonephritis

Immune disorders (transfusion reactions, transplant rejection)

Metabolic diseases (hypercalcemia, hypokalemia, hyperuricemia)

Neoplasm (lymphoma, leukemia, multiple myeloma)

Vascular (sickle cell disease, arteriolar nephrosclerosis, shock)

Crush injuries with myoglobinuria

Burns

Approach to Diagnostic Imaging

■ 1. Ultrasound

- Demonstrates nonspecific pattern of bilateral large, smooth kidneys and excludes obstruction as a cause for oliguria or anuria

Tubulointerstitial Nephritis (Chronic)

Presenting Signs and Symptoms

Progressive insidious renal failure

Common Causes

Drug-induced (analgesics, especially aspirin and phen-
acetin)
Obstructive uropathy
Chronic pyelonephritis
Immune disorders (transplant rejection)
Metabolic diseases (nephrocalcinosis/nephrolithiasis,
oxalosis, cystinosis, gout, diabetes mellitus)
Inherited multisystem disorders (polycystic disease,
multicystic kidney disease, medullary sponge kidney,
sickle cell disease, hereditary nephritis)
Malignancy (multiple myeloma)

Approach to Diagnostic Imaging

■ 1. Ultrasound

- Demonstrates nonspecific pattern of bilateral small,
  smooth kidneys

Cancer of the Urinary Bladder

Presenting Signs and Symptoms

Hematuria, pyuria, frequency, dysuria, and burning

Predisposing Factors

Aniline dyes
Rubber and plastics manufacturing chemicals
Tobacco tars (excretory products)
Schistosomiasis
Bladder calculi (irritative effects)
Bladder exstrophy

Approach to Diagnostic Imaging

■ 1. Excretory urography

- May detect tumors >1.5 cm as irregular filling defects, but is less sensitive than cystoscopy

 Caveat: Cystoscopic biopsy is required for histologic confirmation of the diagnosis.

Staging

■ 1. Magnetic resonance imaging

- Superior to CT for predicting the depth of bladder wall invasion (high-signal tumor disruption of the normally low-signal bladder wall on T2-weighted images)
- Equal to or better than CT for showing tumor extension into the perivesical fat (low-signal tumor versus high-signal fat on T1-weighted images)

■ 2. Computed tomography

- Alternative procedure for staging if MRI is not available (although not as good as MRI for differentiating superficial noninvasive tumors from those invading the bladder muscle)
- Superior to US for defining the pelvic structures and delineating enlargement of paraaortic lymph nodes

Neurogenic Bladder

Presenting Signs and Symptoms

Partial or complete urinary retention
Incontinence
Predisposition to infection and calculus formation

Common Causes

Acute spinal cord trauma
Meningomyelocele
Diabetes mellitus
Central nervous system neoplasm (brain or spinal cord)
Cerebrovascular accident
Herniated intervertebral disc
Demyelinating process (multiple sclerosis, amyotrophic
  lateral sclerosis)
Poliomyelitis
Syphilis

Approach to Diagnostic Imaging

■ 1. Excretory urography

- ■ Demonstrates marked thickening of the bladder
  wall, which has an irregular contour due to
  muscular trabeculation

Note: Although US also can show this appearance,
it does not give any indication of the degree of kidney
function.

Bladder Outlet Obstruction

Presenting Signs and Symptoms

Partial or complete urinary retention
Progressive urinary frequency, urgency, and nocturia
   (due to incomplete emptying and rapid refilling of
   the bladder)
Overflow incontinence
Predisposition to infection and calculus formation

Common Causes

Benign prostatic hyperplasia
Prostatic cancer
Bladder neck obstruction (anatomic versus functional)
Acquired bladder neck stricture (traumatic, postsurgical)
Neurogenic bladder

Approach to Diagnostic Imaging

■ **1. Excretory urography**

■ Preferred imaging technique for demonstrating
   the size of the bladder (markedly dilated or
   small and shrunken)

> **Note:** Excretory urography can also provide valuable information concerning the functional status of the upper urinary tracts. Characteristic findings may suggest prostate enlargement or neurogenic bladder. It is insensitive for detecting bladder tumors.

Cystitis

Presenting Signs and Symptoms

Dysuria, frequency, urgency
Hematuria
Suprapubic pain

Common Causes

Infection (bacteria, tuberculosis, schistosomiasis)
Drug-induced (cyclophosphamide)
Radiation

Approach to Diagnostic Imaging

Notes: Radiographic assessment of *women* with lower urinary tract infection is usually of little value and rarely provides information that aids in clinical management.

Because cystitis in *men* is often associated with obstruction of the lower urinary tract, evaluation should be directed at detecting underlying prostatic or urethral pathology.

■ 1. Voiding cystography or excretory urography

- Demonstrates a diffuse scalloped, irregular contour of the bladder wall and a small capacity bladder
- Gas may be detected within the bladder wall in patients with emphysematous cystitis

Urethritis (Gonococcal)

Presenting Signs and Symptoms

Dysuria
Thick, purulent urethral discharge
Primarily affects men

Approach to Diagnostic Imaging

 Caveat: Uncomplicated infections require *no* imaging (indicated only to detect complications of the disease).

■ 1. Retrograde urethrography

- Preferred technique for demonstrating the location, size, length, and number of urethral strictures, as well as periurethral communications (especially when surgery is contemplated)

Note: Retrograde urethrography is also valuable in postoperative assessment, especially in detecting residual or recurrent stenoses.

Addison's Disease

Presenting Signs and Symptoms

Weakness, fatigue, orthostatic hypotension (early)
Increased pigmentation
Weight loss, dehydration, hypotension (late)
Small heart size
Anorexia, nausea and vomiting, diarrhea
Decreased cold tolerance

Common Causes

Autoimmune process (idiopathic atrophy)
Granulomatous process (tuberculosis, histoplasmosis)
Neoplasm (lymphoma, metastases)
Infarction
Hemorrhage

Approach to Diagnostic Imaging

Note: Addison's disease is a clinical diagnosis based on classic signs and symptoms and confirmed by laboratory tests.

■ 1. Plain abdominal radiograph

- May demonstrate adrenal calcification suggesting prior tuberculosis or histoplasmosis

■ 2. Computed tomography

- May demonstrate enlargement of the adrenal glands secondary to lymphoma or metastases
- Idiopathic atrophy results in very small adrenal glands

Adrenal Virilism (Adrenogenital Syndrome)

Presenting Signs and Symptoms

Hirsutism
Male-pattern baldness
Acne
Deepening of the voice
Amenorrhea and uterine atrophy
Decreased breast size
Increased muscularity

Common Causes

Adrenal hyperplasia (infants)
Adrenal adenoma or carcinoma (adults)

Approach to Diagnostic Imaging

■ 1. Computed tomography

- Procedure of choice for demonstrating the underlying adrenal neoplasm or hyperplasia

Primary Aldosteronism (Conn's Syndrome)

Presenting Signs and Symptoms

Hypertension

Hypokalemia

Increased serum and urine aldosterone (radioimmunoassay)

Low plasma renin activity

Common Causes

Hyperfunctioning adrenal adenoma (80%)

Bilateral adrenal hyperplasia (20%)

Approach to Diagnostic Imaging

■ 1. Computed tomography

- ■ Procedure of choice for detecting the adenoma,
  which is usually small (<2 cm)

Note: Intravenous contrast is *not* needed.

Cushing's Syndrome

Presenting Signs and Symptoms

Truncal obesity with prominent supraclavicular and dorsal cervical fat pads ("buffalo hump")

Rounded (moon) facies

Generalized weakness and muscle wasting

Poor wound healing and easy bruising

Hypertension

Osteoporosis

Glucose intolerance

Reduced resistance to infection

Menstrual irregularities

Common Causes

Adrenal hyperplasia (70%)

Pituitary microadenoma (ACTH-secreting)

Nonpituitary ACTH-secreting tumor (usually from lung tumor)

Adrenal adenoma (20%)

Adrenal carcinoma (10%)

Approach to Diagnostic Imaging

■ 1. Computed tomography (abdomen)

- Preferred initial imaging procedure if biochemical tests suggest an adrenal tumor

---

Note: Intravenous contrast is *not* needed.

■ 2. Magnetic resonance imaging (pituitary)

- Procedure of choice for detecting a functioning microadenoma causing adrenal hyperplasia

■ 3. Plain chest radiograph

- Preferred screening study for detecting an underlying ACTH-producing lung tumor

Pheochromocytoma

Presenting Signs and Symptoms

Hypertension (persistent or paroxysmal)
Tachycardia, diaphoresis, postural hypotension, tachypnea, flushing, cold and clammy skin
Severe headache and tremors
Elevated levels of catecholamines and their metabolites

Common Causes

Catecholamine-secreting tumor of chromaffin cells
Adrenal medulla (90%)
Extra-adrenal sites (paraaortic sympathetic chain, organ of Zuckerkandl near the bifurcation of the aorta, urinary bladder)

Approach to Diagnostic Imaging

■ 1. Computed tomography

- Preferred imaging study for detecting tumors (usually >2 cm) involving the adrenal medulla
- If no adrenal mass is found and clinical suspicion remains high, scanning must be extended to include the remainder of the abdomen and pelvis (most extra-adrenal pheochromocytomas lie in the lumbar sympathetic chain)

 Caveat: Intravenous contrast material is unnecessary and could precipitate a hypertensive crisis.

■ 2. Magnetic resonance imaging

- Procedure of choice (if metaiodobenzylguanidine [MIBG] scanning is not available) to search for extra-adrenal pheochromocytomas not found on CT
- The tumor demonstrates extremely bright signal on T2-weighted images, allowing it to stand out from surrounding structures

---

Note: Radionuclide scans using MIBG are highly sensitive for localizing ectopic pheochromocytomas, but this agent is not widely available.

Adrenal Metastases

Presenting Signs and Symptoms

Asymptomatic

Common Primary Tumors

Carcinomas of lung, breast, and kidney
Melanoma
Lymphoma

Approach to Diagnostic Imaging

■ 1. Computed tomography

- Procedure of choice for detecting these relatively common metastatic lesions, which are often large, irregular, and inhomogeneous and invade adjacent structures

 Caveat: Small metastases tend to be homogeneous, well defined, and indistinguishable from benign adenomas. In addition, even in patients with known primary malignancy, more than 50% of small adrenal masses are benign adrenal lesions and not metastases.

- Low density of a small, homogeneous adrenal mass on unenhanced CT allows a confident diagnosis of an adenoma
- Analysis of the density of an adrenal mass over time (CT washout curve) may allow a confident diagnosis of an adenoma on a contrast-enhanced study
- Percutaneous biopsy may still be required for high-density adrenal masses

■ 2. Magnetic resonance imaging

- Metastases have a higher signal intensity than benign adenomas on T2-weighted sequences
- Metastases show greater enhancement than benign adenomas after gadolinium injection
- On chemical-shift MRI, lipid-laden adenomas have low signal intensity, while metastases have intermediate or high signal
- Chemical-shift imaging is highly accurate for identifying adrenal adenomas without biopsy, although CT-guided biopsy is still required to identify the infrequent adenoma that contains little or no lipid

7

MUSCULOSKELETAL
Donald Resnick

Acute Monarticular Joint Pain

Common Causes

Gout
Calcium pyrophosphate deposition disease (CPPD)
Septic arthritis
Bursitis/tendinitis
Trauma
Hemarthrosis (bleeding diathesis)
Localized manifestation of inflammatory polyarthritis (rheumatoid arthritis, Reiter's syndrome, psoriatic arthritis)

Approach to Diagnostic Imaging

■ 1. Plain skeletal radiograph

- Preferred study for demonstrating soft-tissue swelling and calcification, bone erosions, joint space narrowing, and any underlying fracture

Polyarticular Joint Pain

Common Causes

Rheumatoid arthritis
Ankylosing spondylitis
Reiter's syndrome
Psoriatic arthritis
Osteoarthritis
Systemic lupus erythematosus
Hypertrophic osteoarthropathy
Polymyalgia rheumatica
Diffuse appearance of a usually monarticular condition (gout, CPPD, calcium hydroxyapatite deposition disease, bacterial arthritis)

Approach to Diagnostic Imaging

■ 1. Plain skeletal radiograph

- Preferred study for detecting soft-tissue swelling, calcification, bone erosions, joint space narrowing, and osteophyte formation

Vertebral Collapse (Isolated)

Presenting Signs and Symptoms

Loss of height of an isolated vertebral detected incidentally on a plain chest or abdominal radiograph

Common Causes

Post-menopausal osteopenia
Trauma (old)
Malignancy (metastases, myeloma)

Approach to Diagnostic Imaging

■ 1. Radionuclide bone scan

- Demonstration of focal areas of increased radionuclide uptake (hot spots) at multiple levels is virtually diagnostic of metastases

■ 2. Magnetic resonance imaging

- Diffusely abnormal marrow in an isolated collapsed vertebra indicates a malignant cause (metastases or myeloma); normal marrow or focally abnormal marrow points to a benign etiology (post-menopausal osteopenia or old trauma)

Osteomalacia

Presenting Signs and Symptoms

Diffuse skeletal pain and bony tenderness

Bowing of long bones and loss of height of vertebral bodies (due to weight-bearing on progressively weakened bones)

Common Causes

Vitamin D deficiency (lack of sunlight, dietary deficiency, or malabsorption due to chronic pancreatic insufficiency, gastrectomy, or malabsorption syndrome)

Abnormal metabolism of vitamin D (anticonvulsant therapy, chronic liver disease)

Kidney disease (chronic renal failure, renal tubular acidosis, Fanconi's syndrome)

Chronic administration of aluminum-containing antacids

Tumor-induced

Approach to Diagnostic Imaging

■ 1. Plain skeletal radiograph

- ■ May demonstrate osteopenia (particularly in the spine, pelvis, and lower extremities) with accentuation or indistinctness of secondary trabeculae, thinning of the cortices, and insufficiency fractures (lucent lines running perpendicular to the long axis of the bone)

Osteoporosis

Presenting Signs and Symptoms

Often asymptomatic

Dull aching pain in the bones (particularly in the lower thoracic and lumbar area)

Tendency to develop compression fractures of the vertebrae with minimal or no trauma

Kyphosis of the thoracic spine

Fractures at other sites (hip, wrist) with less trauma than required in normal patients

Common Causes

PRIMARY

Postmenopausal/senile

SECONDARY (<5%)

Endocrine dysfunction

Drug-induced (e.g., steroids)

Prolonged immobilization

Chronic renal failure

Osteogenesis imperfecta

Leukemia

Approach to Diagnostic Imaging

■ 1. Plain radiograph (spine)

- May detect anterior wedging of vertebral bodies (especially in the lower thoracic and upper lumbar regions) and associated ballooning of intervertebral disc spaces, characteristic of compression fractures

Caveat: Plain radiographs of the spine are otherwise of little value because abnormal radiolucency cannot be accurately diagnosed until at least 50–70% of bone substance has been lost.

■ 2. Measurements of bone mineral content

- Various methods (quantitative CT, single- and dual-photon absorptiometry, dual-energy x-ray absorptiometry) are available to assess the quantity of bone in the spine both for initial diagnosis and for following the response to therapy
- There is much debate concerning which imaging method is superior and even whether or not knowing the bone mineral content is clinically more helpful than mere knowledge of a patient's age and sex (in itself fairly accurate for predicting bone-mass quantity)

Note: Most authors agree that knowing the axial bone mineral measurement does *not* help predict which patients are at risk for developing hip and vertebral body fractures, and especially fractures at extra-axial locations.

Ankylosing Spondylitis

Presenting Signs and Symptoms

Recurrent back pain (often nocturnal)

Morning stiffness (usually relieved by activity)

Kyphosis (flexed posture typically eases back pain and paraspinal muscle spasm)

Chest pain and diminished chest expansion (from diffuse costovertebral involvement)

Peripheral joint pain (especially hip or shoulder)

Cauda equina syndrome

Acute iritis (anterior uveitis) in 30%

Constitutional symptoms of fever, fatigue, anorexia, weight loss, and anemia (may be severe)

Primarily affects men (3:1), especially between ages 20 and 40

Approach to Diagnostic Imaging

■ 1. Plain skeletal radiograph

- Earliest finding is erosion and sclerosis involving the sacroiliac joints (especially the iliac side) in a symmetric fashion

- Characteristic abnormalities include squaring of vertebral bodies, syndesmophyte formation, and paraspinal ligamentous calcification that eventually produce the classic "bamboo spine"

■ 2. Computed tomography or magnetic resonance imaging

- Transverse imaging occasionally allows diagnosis when routine radiographs are normal

- Helpful in cases complicated by spinal fracture or arachnoid diverticula

Calcium Pyrophosphate Deposition Disease (CPPD or Pseudogout)

Presenting Signs and Symptoms

Acute attack of pain, swelling, redness, and warmth of one or more joints (especially the knee) in about 25%

Chronic progressive degenerative changes in multiple joints (at times with intermittent acute attacks)

Most patients are asymptomatic, and the condition is very common in persons older than 70 years of age

Approach to Diagnostic Imaging

■ 1. Plain skeletal radiograph

- May demonstrate characteristic calcification of articular cartilage and menisci (chondrocalcinosis) in the knee, triangular fibrocartilage of the wrist, and the symphysis pubis and acetabular region

- May show structural joint changes that resemble osteoarthritis but occur in sites not typically involved in osteoarthritis (glenohumeral joints, wrists, and patellofemoral joints) and are more severe

Gout

Presenting Signs and Symptoms

Acute gouty arthritis is an exquisitely painful monarthritis that typically involves the metatarsophalangeal joint of the big toe (podagra) but also commonly involves the instep, ankle, knee, wrist, and elbow (may be precipitated by minor trauma, overindulgence in food or alcohol, surgery, fatigue, emotional stress, infection, or vascular occlusion)

Chronic gout is characterized by tophaceous deposits of urate crystals in joints, walls of bursae, and tendon sheaths that may lead to chronic joint symptoms, permanent erosive changes, and joint deformity

Increased serum urate concentration and hyperuricemia

Nephrolithiasis

Approach to Diagnostic Imaging

■ 1. Plain skeletal radiograph

- In chronic or recurrent disease, may demonstrate characteristic well defined "rat-bite" erosions with sclerotic borders and overhanging edges (especially in the first metatarsophalangeal joints) with osteoporosis or soft-tissue tophaceous deposits (especially about the elbow, patella, and hand)

■ 2. Magnetic resonance imaging

- Pattern of disease varies, but regions of persistent low signal intensity are characteristic

Neuropathic Arthropathy (Charcot Joint)

Presenting Signs and Symptoms

Rapidly progressive destructive process with effusion, subluxation, and instability of affected joints

Pain is often absent or less severe than would be expected from the degree of joint destruction

"Bag of bones" appearance of involved joint (due to repeated fractures and bony metaplasia that produce free fragments of cartilage or bone)

Precise site of involvement depends on underlying disorder

Common Causes

Diabetes mellitus (foot, spine)

Tabes dorsalis (knee and hip)

Syringomyelia (upper extremity, especially elbow and shoulder)

Spina bifida with meningomyelocele

Leprosy

Quadriplegia

Coma

Approach to Diagnostic Imaging

■ 1. Plain skeletal radiograph

- May demonstrate extensive destructive changes and heterotopic new bone formation

Osteoarthritis

Presenting Signs and Symptoms

Insidious onset and gradual progression of pain that typically involves one or only a few joints, increases with exercise, and may become worse at night or with weather changes

Primary osteoarthritis typically involves weight-bearing joints (hips, knees) and frequently used joints (fingers)

Secondary osteoarthritis is due to a predisposing factor (trauma, congenital abnormality, metabolic disorder) and may be unilateral, appear at an early age, or involve joints that usually are not affected

Stiffness in the morning or after rest (usually brief)

With progressive disease, joints may appear enlarged, motion becomes limited, flexion contractures and subluxations may develop, and tenderness and crepitus may occur

Approach to Diagnostic Imaging

■ 1. Plain skeletal radiograph

- Demonstrates the typical findings of irregular or asymmetric joint space narrowing, hypertrophic bone formation (osteophytes) at the periphery of joints, subchondral sclerosis (increased opacity), and subchondral pseudocysts (geodes)

Note: In the hands, osteoarthritis primarily involves the distal and proximal interphalangeal joints. In the wrist, the disease affects the joints at the base of the thumb. In the knee, the medial portion of the joint is more severely involved in men.

Psoriatic Arthritis

Presenting Signs and Symptoms

Joint abnormalities in about 5% of patients with skin or nail disease

Approach to Diagnostic Imaging

■ 1. Plain skeletal radiograph

- Demonstrates characteristic proliferative erosions (usually affecting the distal and proximal interphalangeal joints of the fingers and toes), as well as possible resorption of terminal phalanges, bony ankylosis, or arthritis mutilans (aggressive, destructive form of the disease)
- May be associated with spondylitis, sacroiliitis, or both (even in the absence of peripheral arthritis)

Reiter's Syndrome

Presenting Signs and Symptoms

Urethritis
Conjunctivitis
Peripheral arthritis
Mucocutaneous lesions (small painless superficial ulcers)

Approach to Diagnostic Imaging

■ 1. Plain skeletal radiograph

- Demonstrates asymmetric, polyarticular proliferative erosions, typically involving the lower
  extremities (especially the toes and the heels)
- May be associated with sacroiliac involvement
  (leading to back pain), which may have a
  unilateral distribution

Rheumatoid Arthritis

Presenting Signs and Symptoms

Symmetric polyarthritis of peripheral joints (especially in the hand, wrist, and foot) with pain, tenderness, and swelling

Typically insidious and progressive joint involvement

Morning stiffness

Rheumatoid nodules (in 30–40% of patients)

Deformities (particularly flexion contractures and ulnar deviation of the fingers)

Carpal tunnel syndrome (due to synovitis of the wrist)

Serum rheumatoid factor

Primarily affects women (3:1) between ages 25 and 50

Approach to Diagnostic Imaging

■ 1. Plain radiograph (hands, wrists, feet)

- Demonstrates the characteristic appearance of soft-tissue swelling, periarticular demineralization, joint space narrowing, and marginal erosions that symmetrically involve the wrists and hands (primarily the metacarpophalangeal and proximal interphalangeal joints)

- Similar findings at the metatarsophalangeal joints of the feet

Note: The "rheumatoid variants" (psoriatic and Reiter's arthritis) more commonly are *asymmetric* and may involve the *distal* interphalangeal joints.

Osteomyelitis (Direct Seeding or Contiguous Spread)

Presenting Signs and Symptoms

Pain and fever with tenderness and soft-tissue swelling

Common Causes

Trauma (open fracture, surgical reduction of closed fracture, penetrating trauma)

Bacterial contamination of orthopedic prosthesis during surgery

Diabetic or atherosclerotic arterial insufficiency of lower extremities (spread from cutaneous foot ulcer)

Sinus or dental infection (osteomyelitis of skull)

Approach to Diagnostic Imaging

■ 1. Plain skeletal radiograph

- May demonstrate bony destruction with the formation of lucent areas, radiopaque sequestra (foci of devitalized bone), and involucra
- An infected prosthesis may show characteristic lucent areas within the shaft of the bone adjacent to the cement about the prosthesis (may also be seen with simple loosening or to particle disease accompanying the breakdown of prosthetic components)

■ 2. Computed tomography

- Indicated to detect sequestra, which usually indicate the need for surgical removal rather than antibiotics alone (as avascular sequestra will not be effectively treated with parenteral medication)

 Caveat: Radionuclide bone scan is of little value because the isotope accumulates in many noninfectious conditions, such as fracture sites, uninfected nonunion of fractures, periosteal new bone, overlying cellulitis, neuropathic arthropathy, and aseptic loosening of prostheses.

■ 3. Magnetic resonance imaging

- Sensitive (but not specific) for detecting osteomyelitis
- Diagnostic difficulty occurs owing to the presence of bone marrow edema (neighborhood reaction) in cases of adjacent soft-tissue infection

Osteomyelitis (Hematogenous)

Presenting Signs and Symptoms

Pain and fever with tenderness and soft-tissue swelling

In *children,* most commonly involves the long bones (especially near the physeal plate at the end of the shaft)

In *adults,* usually affects the vertebral bodies and pelvic bones

Common Causes

Intravenous drug abuse

Hemodialysis

Debilitating diseases

Approach to Diagnostic Imaging

■ 1. Plain skeletal radiograph.

- Although neither sensitive nor specific, their low cost, ready availability, and ability to exclude other diseases that can produce similar symptoms (fractures, tumors) argue for their continued use as the initial evaluation.

■ 2. Radionuclide bone scan

- Demonstrates increased activity early in the disease (evidence of bone destruction on plain skeletal radiographs usually does not appear for at least 1 week and at least 30% of bone destruction is required before osteomyelitis becomes radiographically apparent)
- Permits whole-body imaging when symptoms cannot be localized

 Caveat: Bone scans may take months to normalize after a bone infection becomes sterile, and thus it may be impossible to distinguish a chronic infection of bone from normal healing.

■ 3. Magnetic resonance imaging

- Equally sensitive as (or even more sensitive than) bone scintigraphy for detecting hematogenous osteomyelitis and more specific. It is preferred to radionuclide bone scanning when the signs and symptoms can be localized.
- Repeat imaging with MRI should be considered in all patients who do not improve clinically after 48 h of systemic antibiotic therapy
- Inherent high spatial resolution allows exact anatomic detail that may be valuable for surgical planning

Note: CT has a limited role in the early diagnosis of osteomyelitis.

Osteomyelitis (Vertebral)

Presenting Signs and Symptoms

Insidious onset and gradual progression of back pain
unrelieved by heat, rest, or analgesics and worsened
by movement
Fever typically is minimal or absent
Tenderness to palpation and percussion over affected
bone
Paravertebral muscle spasm
Guarding and splinting on motion

Approach to Diagnostic Imaging

■ 1. Radionuclide bone scan

- Demonstrates increased activity early in the disease (evidence of bone destruction on plain
skeletal radiographs usually does not appear
for at least 1 week)

 Caveat: Increased radionuclide uptake may
be impossible to distinguish from that occurring
with tumors and fractures.

■ 2. Magnetic resonance imaging

- ■ Sensitive for demonstrating a focal abnormal signal intensity in the bone marrow, but does not accurately distinguish between infection and tumor
- ■ Can effectively reveal the full extent of soft-tissue involvement (as can CT)

Note: Plain radiographs of the spine are not sensitive for detecting vertebral osteomyelitis. However, the findings of vertebral body destruction and rapid loss of the adjacent intervertebral disc are highly suggestive of the diagnosis of bacterial infection (as they are uncommon in cases of tumor).

■ 3. Computed tomography

- ■ Although not as accurate in the evaluation of spinal osteomyelitis, contrast-enhanced CT is superb for identifying soft-tissue infections and abscesses

Osteomyelitis (Diabetic Foot)

Note: Osteomyelitis in the diabetic foot represents a diagnostic challenge. The diabetic foot is prone to infection and poor healing due to the decreased blood supply secondary to diabetic vasculopathy, decreased immune response, and repetitive trauma from diabetic neuropathy. Radiographically, the diabetic foot has many features mimicking infection, including bone destruction, debris, and subluxation.

Approach to Diagnostic Imaging

■ 1. Magnetic resonance imaging

- High sensitivity and specificity for evaluation of osteomyelitis in these patients

Note: In diabetic patients, radionuclide bone scan often has abnormal findings even without osteomyelitis.

Infectious Arthritis (Septic Joint)

Presenting Signs and Symptoms

Acute joint pain associated with warmth, tenderness, swelling, and effusion

Fever, chills

Leukocytosis

May be little systemic or local response in patients receiving antiinflammatory drugs

Approach to Diagnostic Imaging

■ 1. Plain skeletal radiograph

- Neither sensitive nor specific, but may demonstrate joint effusion, joint space narrowing, and erosive changes

> **Note:** The diagnosis of infectious arthritis requires a high index of suspicion (especially in patients with underlying chronic joint disease). Therefore, even the remote possibility that a joint might be septic demands aspiration of synovial fluid and a search for the infecting organism by Gram stain and culture (even if plain radiographs are completely normal).

■ 2. Magnetic resonance imaging or radionuclide bone scan

- Not specific, but permits early diagnosis in a patient with a high likelihood of joint infection

■ 3. Ultrasound

- Recommended if symptoms are referable to the hip to rapidly assess for the presence of an effusion (though it is not specific for infection) and to provide imaging-guided joint aspiration

Skeletal Metastases

Presenting Signs and Symptoms

Most often asymptomatic (discovered during staging procedures)

Back pain

Common Primary Tumors

Lung

Breast

Prostate

Thyroid

Kidney

Lymphoma

Melanoma

Approach to Diagnostic Imaging

■ 1. Radionuclide bone scan

- Preferred screening technique for detecting asymptomatic skeletal metastases, which appear as focal areas of increased radionuclide uptake (hot spots)

> **Note:** False-negative results may occur if there is uniform, symmetric uptake of radionuclide by diffuse metastases ("superscan"). The proper diagnosis should be suggested by decreased or no labeling of the kidneys (all radionuclide taken up by skeletal structures so that little or none remains to be excreted by the usual renal route).

■ 2. Plain skeletal radiograph

- If the radionuclide scan is equivocal, plain films should be obtained to confirm that a hot spot represents a metastasis rather than one of the many benign processes that can also cause increased uptake (e.g., infection, degenerative disease, trauma)

- Generally *not* indicated if there are multiple focal radionuclide scan abnormalities involving the axial skeleton that are virtually pathognomonic of metastases

 Caveat: *Never* order a "skeletal survey" to screen for metastases. Plain radiographs are insensitive (40–80% of cancellous bone must be destroyed before a lesion is apparent on these films). However, such surveys are useful in cases of multiple myeloma.

■ 3. Computed tomography or magnetic resonance imaging

- Indicated to evaluate nonspecific focal abnormality on radionuclide scan or specific symptomatic areas that cannot be demonstrated or adequately characterized on plain radiographs

 Caveat: Neither CT nor MRI should ever be used as the initial screening test for suspected skeletal metastases, although either may be used to further define a symptomatic region of the body in a patient with a known primary malignant tumor. With the increasing availability of higher-strength magnets and new computer programs, total body MRI may become an alternative screening test for skeletal metastases.

Multiple Myeloma

Presenting Signs and Symptoms

Persistent unexplained skeletal pain (especially in the back or thorax)

Pathologic fractures and vertebral collapse

Renal failure

Recurrent bacterial infections (especially pneumococcal pneumonia)

Anemia with weakness and fatigue

Hypercalcemia

Excess immunoglobulins

Bence Jones protein

Approach to Diagnostic Imaging

■ 1. Plain skeletal radiograph

- Demonstrates either diffuse osteoporosis or multiple discrete osteolytic ("punched-out") lesions (due to replacement by expanding plasma cell tumors or elaboration of an osteoclast-stimulating factor); these lesions are often associated with pathologic fractures or vertebral collapse

- Diffuse changes may be difficult to recognize unless thinning and expansion of the cortices are appreciated

■ 2. Magnetic resonance imaging

- Preferred imaging study for showing the characteristic diffuse marrow abnormalities (low-intensity tumor replaces normal high-intensity marrow fat on T1-weighted images)
- Can demonstrate compression of the spinal cord secondary to vertebral collapse

 Caveat: Radionuclide bone scan is *not* indicated as a screening test for multiple myeloma because the process is primarily osteolytic with little bone production (thus radionuclide scans typically are falsely normal).

Osteoid Osteoma

Presenting Signs and Symptoms

Pain that classically is worse at night and relieved by
small doses of aspirin

Almost always in patients younger than 30 years

Approach to Diagnostic Imaging

▪ 1. Plain skeletal radiograph

- ▪ May demonstrate the characteristic appearance of
  a small radiolucent zone (nidus) surrounded by
  a large sclerotic zone (reactive bone)

▪ 2. Radionuclide bone scan

- ▪ Indicated if plain film findings cannot distinguish
  osteoid osteoma from osteomyelitis

Note: Because the nidus is extremely vascular, it
avidly accumulates the radionuclide, producing the typical "double-density" sign representing an area of avid
radionuclide uptake (nidus) surrounded by a region of
moderately increased uptake (reactive bone). This is in
contrast to the central photopenic area of osteomyelitis
that represents an avascular focus of purulent material.

■ 3. Computed tomography

- Indicated to define the exact location of the nidus (if not clearly seen on plain films) prior to surgery (because removal of the nidus usually results in complete cessation of pain)

 Caveat: MRI findings in osteoid osteoma include extensive marrow and soft-tissue edema resembling those of a malignant tumor or osteomyelitis.

Primary Malignant Tumors of Bone

Presenting Signs and Symptoms

Pain, soft-tissue mass

Common Types

Osteosarcoma, fibrosarcoma, chondrosarcoma, Ewing's sarcoma

Approach to Diagnostic Imaging

■ 1. Plain skeletal radiograph

- Preferred initial imaging study for demonstrating a lesion's site and appearance (which combined with a patient's age may permit a specific diagnosis)

Note: If a single lesion is detected that could represent a metastasis, a radionuclide bone scan (*not* a plain-film skeletal survey) is essential to detect any other clinically silent lesions.

 Caveat: Although plain radiographic signs may aid in distinguishing benign from malignant lesions, none is infallible, and a biopsy may be required.

■ 2. Magnetic resonance imaging

- Best imaging modality for determining the bony and soft-tissue extent of a lesion (required prior to surgical resection)

 Caveat: The ability of MRI to distinguish benignity from malignancy is controversial, and it may be impossible to determine whether high signal radiating from involved bone in some imaging sequences represents soft-tissue edema or tumor spread.

Soft-Tissue Tumor of Extremity

Presenting Signs and Symptoms

Asymptomatic (incidentally noted either by the patient or an examining physician)

Variety of clinical manifestations, depending on the site and type of lesion

Common Causes

Lipoma

Melanoma

Liposarcoma

Malignant fibrous histiocytoma

Approach to Diagnostic Imaging

■ 1. Plain skeletal radiograph

- Neither sensitive nor specific, but usually performed initially to demonstrate the soft-tissue lesion, its effect on the underlying bone, and any associated calcification

■ 2. Computed tomography or magnetic resonance imaging

- Most accurate imaging procedures for defining the extent of a soft-tissue mass and its relationship to adjacent structures

 Caveat: Although these techniques can sometimes suggest the nature of a soft-tissue neoplasm (especially those containing fat), a biopsy is generally required to determine the precise histologic diagnosis. Intravenous gadolinium is helpful in distinguishing between fluid and solid masses.

■ 3. Ultrasound

- Imaging modality of choice for determining whether a superficial soft-tissue mass thought to represent a cyst is truly fluid-filled

■ 4. Arteriography

- May be indicated as a preoperative study to determine the vascular anatomy
- May be helpful in localizing an area within the mass that will most likely yield accurate biopsy data (the most malignant sites tend to have the greatest vascularity)

Pathologic Fracture

Presenting Signs and Symptoms

Evidence of a fracture following a trivial injury or without a history of trauma

Concomitant evidence of preexisting abnormality (angular deformity, painless swelling, or generalized bone pain)

Common Causes

Malignant neoplasms

Metastases

Benign lesions (e.g., simple bone cyst, enchondroma, giant cell tumor)

Osteoporosis

Approach to Diagnostic Imaging

■ 1. Plain skeletal radiograph

- Preferred initial study for demonstrating that the fracture line traverses a large area of bone destruction or that adjacent or distant bones are riddled with additional lesions

 Caveat: If the underlying lesion is small, the fracture itself may obscure the abnormal lytic or sclerotic area (especially if there is displacement at the fracture site).

■ 2. Computed tomography or magnetic resonance imaging

- May be useful for detecting more subtle indications of underlying abnormal bone

Hip Fracture

Presenting Signs and Symptoms

History of fall with inability or significant difficulty in weight bearing on involved extremity

Pain and bruising in hip region

Common Causes

Trauma

Osteoporosis

Approach to Diagnostic Imaging

■ 1. Plain skeletal radiograph

- Provides definite diagnosis of fracture in the vast majority of cases
- Angled projection may be necessary to demonstrate nondisplaced fracture of the femoral neck

■ 2. Magnetic resonance imaging

- Highly sensitive for detecting radiographically occult fracture
- Indicated if there is a high clinical suspicion of fracture despite normal plain films

■ 3. Radionuclide bone scan

- If MRI is not available, can be used to detect or exclude occult fracture in patient with a high clinical suspicion despite negative plain films
- Because false-negative results may occur in a small percentage of patients (especially the elderly) during the first 72 h after fracture, a repeat scan may be required to reliably exclude a fracture

Pelvic Fracture

Presenting Signs and Symptoms

History of major trauma to pelvis
Pain and bruising in the pelvic region
Substantial internal blood loss
Hematuria

Common Cause

Trauma

Approach to Diagnostic Imaging

■ 1. Plain skeletal radiograph

- Provides definite diagnosis of fracture in most cases (without the need to move the patient, who may have suffered multiple injuries)
- Oblique and angled views (inlet, outlet, Judet) may be required to diagnose or exclude minor fracture
- Second fractures are typical

 Caveat: Sacral foramina fractures may be difficult to detect.

■ 2. Computed tomography

- Indicated if there is a high clinical suspicion of fracture despite normal plain films
- Especially valuable for detecting occult sacral fractures, as well as bone fragments in the hip joint associated with an acetabular fracture
- Can demonstrate hemorrhage and soft-tissue injuries that often occur in conjunction with pelvic fractures

■ 3. Magnetic resonance imaging

- May reveal marrow edema about the fracture site (although the fracture line itself is better seen with CT)

Note: In patients with massive hemorrhage, arteriography may be required to identify the bleeding site and permit transcatheter embolization therapy. Retrograde urethrography and cystography are indicated in fractures of the anterior pelvis to exclude injury to the posterior urethra and bladder.

Scaphoid Fracture

Presenting Signs and Symptoms

Pain in the region of the anatomic snuff-box
High incidence of complications (delayed union, nonunion, avascular necrosis)

Approach to Diagnostic Imaging

■ 1. Plain skeletal radiograph

- Preferred initial study (although it fails to detect
  up to 25% of nondisplaced fractures)
- Delayed radiographs (after 1–2 weeks of immobilization) often demonstrate "initially occult"
  fractures because of resorption and better
  demarcation around the fracture line

■ 2. Magnetic resonance imaging

- High sensitivity for detecting fractures not evident
  on initial plain radiographs
- Enables early diagnosis and definitive treatment
  (decreases risk of complications)
- Acute fractures have decreased signal intensity
  of the proximal pole of T1-weighted images
  and increased signal on T2-weighted and
  fat-suppression sequences
- Avascular necrosis classically has low signal
  intensity on all sequences
- Gadolinium-enhanced sequences may be of value
  in selecting patients with acute fractures who
  are likely to develop avascular necrosis or
  delayed union, as well as in assessing surgical
  eligibility in those with established nonunion
  or avascular necrosis

■ 3. Radionuclide bone scan

- Traditionally considered the imaging modality of choice for early diagnosis of occult fractures (high sensitivity, with optimal imaging at 48 h after injury)
- Similar findings of increased uptake can be seen in disuse states, ligamentous injuries, and reflex sympathetic dystrophy
- Lack of spatial resolution may necessitate further imaging studies (CT, MRI) for more precise anatomic information prior to definitive treatment
- Negative bone scan virtually excludes the possibility of scaphoid or other occult fracture

Stress Fracture

Presenting Signs and Symptoms

Activity-related pain relieved by rest (typically associated with the repetition of a new or different strenuous activity)

Localized tenderness and soft-tissue swelling

Common Examples

March fracture (metatarsals in military recruits)

Lower extremity fractures in athletes, joggers, and dancers

Approach to Diagnostic Imaging

■ 1. Plain skeletal radiograph

- May demonstrate a radiolucent line or a band of sclerosis associated with periosteal and endosteal thickening

Caveat: Plain radiographic evidence of a stress fracture may not be detectable for several weeks.

■ 2. Radionuclide bone scan

- Sensitive for early detection of a stress fracture
- May be impossible to differentiate shin splint from early stress fracture (treated differently)
- Triple-phase technique should be used to maximize specificity

■ 3. Magnetic resonance imaging

- Extremely sensitive for detecting stress injuries and may prove to be more specific than radionuclide scanning
- Usually reserved for cases in which radiographic findings are indeterminate
- In early stress fractures, the marrow has low signal intensity on T1-weighted images and has progressively higher intensity with increased T2-weighting
- Fat-saturation techniques are especially useful, with the increased water content of the associated medullary edema or hemorrhage resulting in high signal intensity against the dark background of suppressed fat
- Fracture line may not be seen

Meniscal Tear (Knee)

Presenting Signs and Symptoms

Pain and swelling
Click in movement of the joint
Knee "giving way" or locking in a single position

Approach to Diagnostic Imaging

■ 1. Magnetic resonance imaging

- Imaging procedure of choice for detecting partial and complete meniscal tears, as well as associated abnormalities of the collateral and cruciate ligaments

Note: Arthrography of the knee is almost obsolete.

 Caveat: The need for both MRI and arthroscopy is controversial. Some studies have indicated that arthroscopy alone is sufficient and financially advisable, except perhaps in instances of recurrent knee pain following previous meniscal surgery or repair.

Rotator Cuff Tear

Presenting Signs and Symptoms

Pain when the arm is raised above the shoulder or adducted across the chest, but not when the arm is held down by the side

Weakness of shoulder abduction (due to underuse atrophy of the deltoid)

Approach to Diagnostic Imaging

■ 1. Magnetic resonance imaging (shoulder)

- Rapidly becoming the imaging procedure of choice for detecting partial and complete rotator cuff tears
- Noninvasive and does not require the technical expertise required for shoulder arthrography

Note: The imaging workup is based on the needs of the orthopedic surgeon. If all that is needed is the detection of full-thickness tears of the rotator cuff (as opposed to partial-thickness tears), arthrography of the glenohumeral joint may be sufficient.

■ 2. Ultrasound

- Sensitive for diagnosing rotator cuff tear, but requires considerable examiner expertise

Child Abuse

Presenting Signs and Symptoms

Nonaccidental intracranial and skeletal injuries (due to direct blows or shaking)

Most commonly involves children younger than age 2

May be bruises, seizures, coma, lethargy, retinal hemorrhage, shallow respirations

Approach to Diagnostic Imaging

■ 1. Plain radiographs (skeletal survey)

- Demonstrates multiple fractures of varying age or unusual fractures
- Injuries highly specific for child abuse include metaphyseal (corner) fractures and fractures of the posterior ribs, sternum, scapula, and spinous processes
- Less specific injuries include epiphyseal injuries, complex skull fractures, and fractures of the vertebral bodies, metacarpals, and metatarsals
- Fractures of the clavicle and the shafts of long bones also are common

■ 2. Computed tomography or magnetic resonance imaging

- Indicated if there is a complex skull fracture or clinical evidence of intracranial injury to detect subdural hematoma, cortical contusion, shearing injury, or subarachnoid hemorrhage

■ 3. Radionuclide bone scan

- May be effective to survey the entire skeleton, although metaphyseal fractures may be missed

---

Note: There is generally *no* indication for any other imaging study.

Avascular Necrosis

Presenting Signs and Symptoms

Pain (most commonly affecting the hip or knee, although the ankle, shoulder, and elbow also may be involved)

Common Causes

Trauma
Steroid therapy
Alcoholism
Pancreatitis
Collagen vascular diseases
Sickle cell disease and other hemoglobinopathies
Renal transplantation
Infiltrative diseases (e.g., Gaucher's disease)
Caisson's disease ("the bends")
Legg-Calvé-Perthes disease

Approach to Diagnostic Imaging

■ 1. Plain skeletal radiograph

- Not sensitive, but ideal for following the disorder from patchy sclerosis and subchondral lucency (thin line beneath the articular surface) to collapse of the articular surface, dense bony sclerosis, and joint fragmentation

■ 2. Magnetic resonance imaging

- Most sensitive study for detecting the earliest changes of avascular necrosis when plain radiographs and radionuclide scans are normal
- In the hip, may demonstrate a characteristic abnormal signal intensity area on some imaging sequences that virtually always involves the anterosuperior portion of the femoral head

3. Radionuclide bone scan

- May show abnormal uptake when plain radiographs are still normal (although not as sensitive as MRI)

Carpal Tunnel Syndrome

Presenting Signs and Symptoms

Pain, paresthesias, and sensory deficits in the distribution of the median nerve

May be weakness or atrophy in the muscles controlling abduction and apposition of the thumb

Positive Tinel's sign (paresthesias after percussion of the median nerve in the volar aspect of the wrist)

Predisposing Factors

Occupations requiring repetitive hand and wrist motion

Gout

Calcium pyrophosphate deposition disease (CPPD)

Acromegaly

Myxedema

Pregnancy

Oral contraceptives

Approach to Diagnostic Imaging

■ 1. Magnetic resonance imaging

- Can show swelling of the median nerve at the proximal carpal tunnel, flattening of the nerve at the distal carpal tunnel, and signal abnormalities within or surrounding the median nerve
- Excellent soft-tissue contrast allows demonstration of subtle soft-tissue changes and mild compression of the median nerve
- Modality of choice for assessing surrounding bony structures

■ 2. Ultrasound

- Suggested as a low-cost alternative to MRI (similar imaging criteria)

■ 3. Computed tomography

- Can assess the fibrous roof of the carpal tunnel and analyze the structures coursing through the canal

Note: CT is of limited value because of the similar attenuation values of the contents of the carpal tunnel.

■ 4. Plain radiograph (wrist)

- Specific radiographic projections (including the carpal tunnel view) can permit an evaluation of the osseous structures bordering the carpal tunnel

Congenital Hip Dislocation

Presenting Signs and Symptoms

Inability to completely abduct the thigh to the surface of
the examining table when the hip and knee are flexed
(Ortolani's sign)

Hip click (audible or palpable "clunk") with abduction
and external rotation of the femur (as the femoral
head reenters the acetabulum)

If unilateral, shortened leg with asymmetric skin creases
in the thigh

Predisposing Factors

Female infants
Breech presentation
Positive family history

Approach to Diagnostic Imaging

Note: Congenital hip dislocation is a *clinical* diagnosis.

■ 1. Plain radiograph (hips)

- Often not diagnostic in the neonatal period, but
  may be of value as a baseline study (to permit
  comparison with subsequent radiographic
  assessment as the child grows and develops)

■ 2. Ultrasound

- Can confirm the clinical diagnosis, even in the neonatal period, with dynamic imaging (counterpart to clinical maneuvers used in physical examination)

■ 3. Magnetic resonance imaging

- May reveal structural abnormalities not evident on routine radiographs

Myasthenia Gravis

Presenting Signs and Symptoms

Ptosis, diplopia, and muscle fatigability after exercise
Dysarthria and dysphagia
Bulbar symptoms (alteration in voice, nasal regurgitation, choking)
Life-threatening respiratory muscle involvement (10%)
Positive edrophonium test

Common Causes

Autoimmune condition associated with thymoma in up to 30% of patients

Note: A larger percentage (up to 50%) of patients with thymoma have or will develop myasthenia gravis.

Approach to Diagnostic Imaging

■ 1. Plain chest radiograph

- Initial imaging procedure for detecting a thymoma, which appears as a smooth or lobulated soft-tissue mass that typically arises near the origin of the great vessels at the base of the heart

■ 2. Computed tomography

- Most sensitive technique for detecting small thymomas not evident on conventional radiographs
- Preferred method for demonstrating local invasion of tumor through thymic capsule to involve pleura, lung, pericardium, chest wall, diaphragm, and great vessels (occurs in 10–15% of patients)

 Caveat: Even CT may be unable to distinguish small thymic tumors from a normal or hyperplastic gland, especially in young patients with a large amount of residual thymic tissue.

Osgood-Schlatter Disease

Presenting Signs and Symptoms

Pain, swelling, and tenderness over the anterior tibial tubercle (at the patellar tendon insertion)

Common Cause

Trauma from excessive traction by the patellar tendon on its immature apophyseal insertion

Approach to Diagnostic Imaging

■ 1. Plain radiograph (knee)

- Demonstrates soft-tissue swelling associated with fragmentation of the anterior tibial tubercle

■ 2. Magnetic resonance imaging

- Often reveals diffuse thickening of the patellar tendon

Paget's Disease

Presenting Signs and Symptoms

Usually asymptomatic (discovered incidentally on radiographs or routine laboratory studies)

Symptoms (typically insidious onset) may include pain, pathologic fracture of weakened bone, deformities, high-output cardiac failure, headaches, decreased hearing, and increasing skull size

Increasingly severe pain suggests fracture or sarcomatous degeneration (1% of patients)

Approach to Diagnostic Imaging

■ 1. Plain skeletal radiograph

- Demonstrates cortical thickening and overall increased density of affected bones, which have an abnormal internal architecture and often show bowing or overgrowth
- Detects pathologic fractures or microfractures (tibia, femur)
- Shows areas of osteolysis in cases of sarcomatous degeneration

■ 2. Radionuclide bone scan

- Most efficient method for screening multiple areas of the skeleton to search for multicentric lesions

Note: MRI and CT are the most accurate imaging modalities in the patient with suspected sarcomatous degeneration of Paget's disease.

Painful Prosthesis

Presenting Signs and Symptoms

Pain in and around the affected joint
Fever, leukocytosis (if infected)

Common Causes

Loosening of prosthesis
Infection
Particle disease related to inflammatory reaction about
polyethylene or cement fragments
Pathologic fracture

Approach to Diagnostic Imaging

■ 1. Plain skeletal radiograph

- Can demonstrate excessive lucency around the
prosthesis, fracture of the prosthesis or adjacent
bone, or prosthesis dislocation

■ 2. Radionuclide bone scan

- Indicated if there is a high clinical suspicion of
loosening or infection despite normal plain
films
- Negative scan makes infection unlikely

Note: If there is clinical suspicion of infection, the
joint is aspirated to obtain fluid for culture.

■ 3. Arthrography

- Can demonstrate loosening by showing gap between prosthesis, cement, and bone when contrast material is injected under pressure
- Analysis and culture of fluid obtained during the procedure can diagnose or exclude infection

■ 4. Magnetic resonance imaging

- Although there is currently no clinical role for MRI in assessing the painful prosthesis containing metal (though it can be used to assess synovitis related to Silastic™ implants), articles have appeared suggesting that technical developments for the use of this modality are under active investigation

Reflex Sympathetic Dystrophy (Sudeck's Atrophy)

Presenting Signs and Symptoms

Pain and tenderness (usually of a hand or foot) associated with vasomotor instability, trophic skin changes, and rapid development of osteopenia

Common Causes

Local trauma
Peripheral nerve injury
Stroke

Approach to Diagnostic Imaging

■ 1. Plain skeletal radiograph

- May demonstrate diffuse or patchy osteopenia of the involved extremity (especially the hands or feet)

■ 2. Radionuclide scan

- Demonstrates diffuse increased uptake in the involved area (but this is nonspecific)
- May show foci of decreased radionuclide uptake in children

Slipped Capital Femoral Epiphysis

Presenting Signs and Symptoms

Insidious onset of hip stiffness that improves with rest

Limp

Hip pain (radiating down the anteromedial thigh to the knee)

In advanced cases, pain on motion of the affected hip, with limited flexion, abduction, and medial rotation

May be associated with chondrolysis and avascular necrosis with epiphyseal collapse (if blood supply is compromised)

Most commonly affects overweight teenagers (usually boys)

Approach to Diagnostic Imaging

■ 1. Plain radiograph (hip)

- ■ Demonstrates widening of the physeal line and/or displacement (posterior and inferior) of the femoral head

 Caveat: Early diagnosis dramatically improves the outcome because treatment becomes more difficult in advanced stages.

8

NEUROLOGIC

Burton P. Drayer

▶ DISORDERS

Coma

Presenting Signs and Symptoms

Sustained state of unconsciousness, defined by the neurological examination primarily in terms of lack of response to external stimuli

Common Causes

Diffuse hypoxic brain injury
Disease of organs other than the brain
  Liver (hepatic encephalopathy)
  Kidney (uremic encephalopathy)
  Lung (hypoxia, carbon dioxide narcosis)
  Pancreas (diabetes, hypoglycemia)
Exogenous poisons (sedatives, narcotics, psychotropic drugs, anticonvulsants, heavy metals)
Acid-base abnormalities affecting the central nervous system
Disordered temperature regulation (hypothermia, heat stroke)
Inflammatory or infiltrative disorders (encephalitis, cerebral vasculitis)
Seizure and post-ictal states

Approach to Diagnostic Imaging

■ 1. Computed tomography or magnetic resonance imaging

- Preferred imaging techniques whenever the cause of coma is unexplained

---

Note: Unless meningitis is suspected and the patient is clinically deteriorating, imaging should *precede* lumbar puncture.

Acute Altered Mental Status

Presenting Signs and Symptoms

Vigorous stimuli required to elicit a response (stupor)
Unarousable unresponsiveness (coma)

Common Causes

Trauma (diffuse cerebral edema; epidural, subdural, intraparenchymal, or subarachnoid hemorrhage)
Anoxia or ischemia (stroke, syncope)
Epilepsy (postictal state)
Exogenous toxins (alcohol, hypnotics, narcotics)
Endogenous toxins (uremia, hepatic coma, diabetic acidosis, hypoglycemia, hyponatremia)
Brain tumor, infarction, abscess, or meningitis

Approach to Diagnostic Imaging

■ 1. Computed tomography

- Can rapidly determine whether there is intracerebral or extracerebral hemorrhage, mass lesion, hydrocephalus, or herniation requiring emergency surgical decompression

 Caveat: Acute brain infarction may not be detected using CT. Nevertheless, CT answers the critical question of whether hemorrhage is present.

■ 2. Magnetic resonance imaging

- Procedure of choice in *subacute* phase for better visualization of the temporal lobes (e.g., herpes encephalitis, neoplasm, vascular malformation), brain stem (e.g., central pontine myelinolysis), white matter (e.g., multiple sclerosis), superior colliculi and mammillary bodies (Wernicke's), and globus pallidus (e.g., hepatic encephalopathy). In general, MRI is the procedure of choice for the diagnosis of any disease affecting the brain.

Note: Plain skull radiographs are of little value and should rarely be obtained.

■ 3. MR or CT angiography

- Both techniques are valuable as the initial procedure for evaluating atherosclerotic, aneurysmal, and veno-occlusive disease, as well as vascular malformations, that involve the aortic arch and the carotid and vertebrobasilar vessels, including the circle of Willis.
- Both MRA and CTA are generally performed after the intravenous administration of contrast material (except for brain MRA)

Amaurosis Fugax

Presenting Sign and Symptom

Ipsilateral blindness that usually resolves fully within 2–30 min (sudden onset and brief duration)

Common Causes

Plaques or atherosclerotic ulcers involving the carotid artery in the neck

Emboli arising from mural thrombi in a diseased heart

Approach to Diagnostic Imaging

■ 1. Magnetic resonance imaging (brain)

- Can evaluate for infarction

■ 2. MR or CT angiography (neck and head)

- Excellent screening study for excluding significant atherosclerotic narrowing and dissection, detecting vascular occlusion, and visualizing the anterior, middle, and posterior cerebral arteries (in addition to the carotid, vertebral, and basilar arteries)

Note: The surgical criteria of 60% stenosis (Asymptomatic Carotid Artery Stenosis Trial [ACAST]) or 70% stenosis (North American Symptomatic Carotid Endarterectomy Trial [NASCET]) can be established using magnetic resonance angiography (MRA) of the neck and head. Although nonenhanced and three-dimensional time-of-flight MRA are excellent, the addition of a rapid bolus infusion of paramagnetic contrast material may improve visualization of the carotid bifurcation and definitely improves visualization of the aortic arch and emerging arterial origins.

■ 3. Duplex, color-flow Doppler ultrasound

- Accurate noninvasive screening study that combines high-resolution, real-time imaging of the carotid arteries with hemodynamic information about blood flow velocity provided by the Doppler technique

---

Note: Other noninvasive tests (ophthalmodynamometry, oculoplethysmography) are not indicated because they cannot accurately detect carotid plaques and ulcerations.

■ 4. Echocardiography

- Indicated to detect mural thrombi in the heart if no carotid lesion has been identified that could explain the patient's symptoms

■ 5. Computed tomography (brain)

- Can evaluate for infarction, but less sensitive than magnetic resonance imaging (MRI)

Aphasia

Presenting Signs and Symptoms

Disorder of language comprehension or production resulting from a cerebral abnormality
  Receptive aphasia (Wernicke's area)
  Conduction aphasia (arcuate fasciculus)
  Expressive aphasia (Broca's area)
May be associated with right hemiparesis (usually due to a cortical lesion in the left middle cerebral artery distribution) or right hemisensory deficit
Must be distinguished from dysarthria, an abnormality of motor speech articulation rather than language, which results from a capsular or brainstem corticospinal tract lesion

Common Causes

Cerebral infarction (dominant hemisphere)
Intracerebral hematoma
Intracerebral neoplasm or abscess (slower, subacute onset)

Approach to Diagnostic Imaging

■ 1. Computed tomography

- Rapidly identifies or excludes intracranial hemorrhage or mass, but cannot definitively exclude acute infarction.
- Remains the "gold standard" for distinguishing acute intracerebral hematoma from cerebral infarction

■ 2. Magnetic resonance imaging

- Routinely perform T1-weighted, intermediate or FLAIR, T2-weighted, gradient echo, and diffusion-weighted pulse sequences
- Highly sensitive for diagnosing acute stroke within 3 h of symptom onset using the diffusion images
- If negative, extremely accurate in excluding acute cerebral infarction
- In rehabilitative phase of chronic infarction causing aphasia, functional MRI may be used to determine if the localization of language function has changed (plasticity)
- Provides improved localization and characterization of any cerebral abnormality detected by CT (e.g., vascular malformation, complicated hemorrhagic process, infarction, mass lesion) and improved specificity for distinguishing the etiology of aphasia

■ 3. MR or CT angiography (neck and head)

- Can often detect the site of a stenosis or occlusion related to acute infarction

 Caveat: Conventional arteriography is indicated *only* if noninvasive studies suggest an underlying aneurysm or arteriovenous malformation *and* a neurointerventional or neurosurgical procedure is seriously being considered.

Ataxia

Presenting Signs and Symptoms

Disorder of stance and gait

Axial signs may predominate (midline cerebellar abnormality)

Appendicular (extremity) signs may predominate (hemispheric cerebellar abnormality)

May have associated tremor, nystagmus, or cranial nerve findings

Must be distinguished from gait apraxia (frontal lobe abnormality) and gait instability related to lower motor neuron disease

Common Causes

Any abnormality involving the cerebellum, cerebellar peduncles, cerebellar pathways in the brain stem, or posterior columns

Common precipitating factors include:

Metabolic secondary to alcohol overuse, anticonvulsant use, the remote effects of cancer (paraneoplastic)

Neurodegenerative (familial cerebellar degeneration, including olivopontocerebellar atrophy, Friedreich's ataxia, and Holmes' cerebellar atrophy)

Neoplasms (commonly medulloblastoma, astrocytoma, and ependymoma in children and metastases and hemangioblastoma in adults)

Demyelinating (multiple sclerosis, acute disseminated encephalomyelitis, progressive multifocal leukoencephalopathy)

Vascular (cerebellar hematoma, infarction, or vascular malformation)

Cysts (arachnoid, epidermoid)

Approach to Diagnostic Imaging

■ 1. Computed tomography

- Procedure of choice in an *acute* case without a history of trauma to exclude an acute intraparenchymal hemorrhage or mass effect on posterior fossa structures

- Less sensitive than MRI for evaluating the posterior fossa because of transverse artifacts from the temporal bones and single axial-plane visualization

■ 2. Magnetic resonance imaging

- Procedure of choice for chronic or progressive gait disturbance

- Nonenhanced study is generally adequate in terms of sensitivity and provides the added benefit of delineating secondary abnormalities (e.g., basal ganglia abnormalities in olivopontocerebellar atrophy, additional lesions in metastases)

- Contrast enhancement may improve specificity (e.g., enhancing peripheral nodule in cystic hemangioblastoma, detection of multiple metastases)

 Caveat: Arteriography is indicated *only* if noninvasive studies suggest an underlying aneurysm or arteriovenous malformation *and* a surgical or interventional radiologic procedure is seriously being considered.

Carotid Bruit (Asymptomatic)

Presenting Signs and Symptoms

Asymptomatic

High-pitched sound heard over the region of the carotid artery bifurcation in the neck (must be distinguished from a venous hum, which is continuous, heard best with the patient sitting or standing, and eliminated by compression of the ipsilateral internal jugular vein)

Common Cause

Narrowing of the lumen of the extracranial carotid artery (usually in the bifurcation region) related to atherosclerotic disease

Approach to Diagnostic Imaging

■ 1. Duplex, color-flow Doppler ultrasound

- Accurate noninvasive screening study that combines high-resolution, real-time imaging of the carotid arteries with hemodynamic information about blood flow velocity provided by the Doppler technique (negative predictive value greater than 99%)

- Should be performed in patients with cervical bruits who are scheduled to undergo major vascular surgery elsewhere (greater than 80% carotid stenosis increases the risk for transient ischemic attack or stroke during surgery)

- About 20% of carotid arteries considered to be completely occluded may still have some lumen patency.

Note: Although some advocate a battery of non-invasive tests, including ophthalmodynamometry and oculoplethysmography, these generally only add unnecessary expense.

■ 2. Magnetic resonance imaging (brain)

- Can evaluate for infarction with standard and diffusion pulse sequences

■ 3. MR or CT angiography (neck and head)

- Excellent screening studies for excluding significant atherosclerotic narrowing, detecting vascular occlusion, and visualizing the vertebral and the anterior, middle, and posterior cerebral arteries, in addition to the carotids

■ 4. Computed tomography (brain)

- Can evaluate for infarction, but less sensitive than MRI

Dementia

Presenting Signs and Symptoms

Permanent or progressive decline in intellectual function (recent memory, concentration, judgment, orientation, ability to speak or read)

Common Causes

Alzheimer's disease (also Pick's disease, frontobasal degeneration)
Multi-infarct (severe)
Metabolic/nutritional/endocrine (including Wernicke–Korsakoff syndrome)
Brain tumor
Chronic central nervous system infection
Normal pressure hydrocephalus
AIDS encephalopathy
Repetitive trauma (e.g., boxers)
Chronic subdural hematoma
Creutzfeldt–Jakob (prion) encephalopathy

Approach to Diagnostic Imaging

■ 1. Magnetic resonance imaging

- Most sensitive for demonstrating large masses, hydrocephalus, and other treatable abnormalities, as well as ischemic white matter disease, small infarctions, Wernicke–Korsakoff syndrome, and primary degenerative dementia

Note: Differentiation of potentially reversible or modifiable causes of dementia from Alzheimer's disease using structural imaging influences patient management during the initial evaluation.

- Increased signal in the globus pallidus and pars reticulate of the substantia nigra on T1-weighted imaging (manganese accumulation or excessive Alzheimer's Type 2 glial protein) is seen with hepatic failure
- Hyperintense signal in the putamen and in the cortex on T2-weighted and diffusion imaging suggests Creutzfeldt-Jakob encephalopathy
- Excellent high-resolution depiction of the temporal lobes without the artifacts inherent in CT

■ 2. Positron emission tomography

- Can be used as an adjunct examination in patients with suspected Alzheimer's or fronto-temporal (Pick's) dementia by defining glucose utilization in the temporal and parietal association areas or fronto-temporal regions

 Caveat: Because brain "atrophy" increases with age in persons with normal mental status, structural MRI and CT imaging may not be a reliable indication of intellectual impairment in the elderly population.

Developmental Disorders

Presenting Signs and Symptoms

Broad spectrum of neurologic deficits

Common Types

Cephaloceles
Chiari malformations
Tuberous sclerosis
Sturge–Weber syndrome
Von Hippel–Lindau disease
Cerebellar dysplasia
Posterior fossa cystic malformations (e.g., Dandy–Walker deformity)
Neurofibromatosis
Holoprosencephaly
Migration disorders (lissencephaly, pachygyria, polymicrogyria, heterotopic gray matter, schizencephaly, abnormalities of the corpus callosum)

Approach to Diagnostic Imaging

■ 1. Magnetic resonance imaging

- Imaging procedure of choice for characterizing and defining the extent of developmental disorders of the CNS
- Ultra high-resolution may be helpful in delineating more subtle cortical abnormalities
- Other advantages include multiplanar imaging and the ability to image the spinal canal as well as the brain

■ 2. Computed tomography

- If the patient is uncooperative and heavy sedation is contraindicated, ease of access and rapid scanning may favor performance of CT
- Useful for follow-up of shunt function by comparing ventricular size

Headache

Common Causes

Increased intracranial pressure (neoplasm, abscess, hemorrhage, meningeal irritation)

Vascular disturbance (migraine, hypertension, cluster headaches)

Toxins (alcoholism, uremia, lead, systemic infection)

Trauma

Extracranial site (disorders of paranasal sinuses, eye, ear, teeth, cervical spine)

Temporal arteritis (in elderly population)

Approach to Diagnostic Imaging

Note: Suggested guidelines for neuroimaging in adult patients with new-onset headache are:

First or worst headache
Increased frequency and increased severity of headache
New-onset headache after age 50
New-onset headache with history of cancer or immunodeficiency
Headache with fever, neck stiffness, and meningeal signs
Headache with abnormal neurological examination

There is no need for neuroimaging in patients with migraine and normal neurologic examination.

■ 1. Magnetic resonance imaging

- Most sensitive technique for detecting cerebral lesions responsible for headache (especially in patients who have coexistent abnormal neurologic signs)
- Imaging evaluation is usually unnecessary in patients with no neurologic abnormalities and who have either continuous headaches of long duration (many months or years) or intermittent recurrent headaches
- If an aneurysm is suspected even though CT is normal, a lumbar puncture and CTA of the head can be performed

 Caveat: Patients with severe *acute* headaches should be imaged with non-contrast head CT because of the suspicion of subarachnoid hemorrhage, acute hydrocephalus, or an enlarging intracranial mass. If meningitis is suspected, a contrast enhanced scan can follow the non-contrast study.

Note: There is *no* indication for conventional skull radiographs. If disease of the paranasal sinuses is suspected, a limited coronal CT study can be performed.

Hearing Loss: Conductive

Sites of Dysfunction

Any process that impedes transmission of sound waves
from the auricle to the oval window

> **Note:** Audiometry and careful clinical examination
> are essential to distinguish conductive from sensori-
> neural hearing loss.

Common Causes

Complete obstruction of external auditory canal
  Congenital atresia or stenosis
  Neoplasm (exostosis)
  Cholesteatoma
  Cerumen impaction
Disorders of tympanic membrane
  Chronic inflammation
  Recurrent inflammation and healing (myringosclerosis)
  Perforation
Disorders of middle ear
  Congenital
  Inflammation and infection (effusion)
  Neoplasm (glomus tympanicum tumor)
  Trauma (ossicular disruption, hemotympanum)

Approach to Diagnostic Imaging

■ 1. Computed tomography

- Thin, high-resolution CT slices demonstrate the location and extent of middle ear neoplasms and other abnormalities
- Contrast-enhanced imaging with soft-tissue algorithms is useful to evaluate extratemporal extension of tumors

■ 2. Magnetic resonance imaging

- Thin-section, T2-weighted images may highlight the presence and extension of inflammatory and neoplastic abnormalities

Hearing Loss: Sensorineural

Sites of Dysfunction

Neuroepithelial hair cells of cochlea (sensory loss)

Neurons of spiral ganglion and central auditory pathways (neural loss)

> **Note:** Hearing loss may have associated vestibular symptomatology. Audiometry and careful clinical examination are essential to distinguish conductive from sensorineural hearing loss.

Common Causes

Congenital (genetic abnormalities, intrauterine exposure to drugs, toxins, infection)

Infection (viral, mumps, syphilis, labyrinthitis ossificans)

Neoplasm (acoustic schwannoma, meningioma, meningeal carcinomatosis, metastasis, epidermoid)

Trauma (cochlear "concussion," fracture through labyrinth or internal auditory canal)

Autoimmune (systemic lupus erythematosus, Wegener's granulomatosis, polyarteritis nodosa, Cogan's syndrome, sarcoidosis)

Vascular (compromise of inner ear blood supply, sickle cell disease)

Metabolic (hypothyroidism, diabetes mellitus)

Multiple sclerosis (brain stem)

Approach to Diagnostic Imaging

TEENAGER/ADULT

▪ 1. Magnetic resonance imaging

- Best modality for demonstrating small tumors, abnormal labyrinth signal intensity, leptomeningeal enhancement, and brain parenchymal disease
- Routine use of thin-section axial and coronal images using T1- and T2-weighted and enhanced T1-weighted images

▪ 2. Computed tomography

- Indicated for patients with trauma or suspicion of labyrinth dysplasia
- Thin-section axial and coronal images using bony algorithms

INFANT/CHILD

▪ 1. Computed tomography

- Preferred modality for showing inner ear dysplasia

 Caveat: Be aware of radiation dosage.

▪ 2. Magnetic resonance imaging

- Indicated for patients with suspected brain parenchymal disease who have a normal CT scan

Hearing Loss: Mixed

Sites of Dysfunction

Combination of sensorineural and conductive hearing loss

Common Causes

Otosclerosis
Osteogenesis imperfecta
Paget's disease
Osteopetrosis (marble-bone disease)
Engelmann's disease (progressive diaphyseal dysplasia)
Pyle's disease (craniometaphyseal dysplasia)

Approach to Diagnostic Imaging

■ 1. Computed tomography

- Thin sections with bone algorithms are employed to detect conductive component
- Contrast-enhanced imaging with soft-tissue algorithms of the internal auditory canal and brain are used to identify sensorineural component

■ 2. Magnetic resonance imaging

- Utilize 3-mm sections in the axial and coronal planes
- Infusion of contrast material is helpful for defining small tumors in the internal auditory canal region and multiple schwannomas

Low Back Pain

Note: One of the major causes for physician visits and the most common reason for work disability. In those with uncomplicated back pain, early treatments are generally aimed at symptomatic relief. In up to 85% of patients, a precise anatomic diagnosis can not be made and the cause is ascribed to some nonspecific muscle strain, ligamentous injury, and spinal degenerative changes.

Approach to Diagnostic Imaging

Note: Imaging is indicated when there is radiculopathy, a suspicion of infection or malignancy, or findings consistent with cauda equina syndrome, a true surgical emergency (see individual sections later in this chapter). Thus, imaging can be safely limited to a minority of patients with low back pain in the primary care setting.

■ 1. Plain skeletal radiograph

- Often the first imaging technique, though of limited value since radiographs cannot directly visualize disks or nerve roots.

■ 2. Magnetic resonance imaging

- Non-enhanced axial and sagittal T1- and T2-weighted images to include the level of the conus constitute the definitive study for detecting the underlying cause of low back pain
- Contrast enhancement is used predominantly to evaluate the postoperative "failed back"

Note: Numerous imaging findings are seen in the spines of asymptomatic patients. These include spinal stenosis, mild scoliosis, transitional vertebra, spondylolysis, Schmorl's nodes, spina bifida occulta, and degenerative changes, all of which are equally prevalent in persons with and without low back pain.

Movement Disorder

Presenting Signs and Symptoms

Parkinsonian symptoms (including bradykinesia, rigidity, tremor)

Common Causes

Parkinson's disease
Huntington's disease

Approach to Diagnostic Imaging

■ 1. Magnetic resonance imaging

- Increased iron in the putamen and caudate (hyperintensity on T2 and T2* images) suggests Parkinson's disease that will not be responsive to drug therapy (multiple system atrophy)
- Excludes a mass or other lesion that may mimic Parkinsonian symptoms

■ 2. Positron emission tomography

- Decreased glucose utilization in the caudate nucleus suggests Huntington's disease

Proptosis

Presenting Signs and Symptoms

Anterior displacement of the globe (exophthalmos)
Redness and irritation of the eye

Common Causes

Trauma
Graves' disease (thyroid ophthalmopathy)
Orbital neoplasm
Orbital inflammatory disease

Approach to Diagnostic Imaging

■ 1. Computed tomography

- Procedure of choice for detecting focal mass, fracture, retrobulbar hematoma, radiopaque foreign body, or abnormality of the globe
- Detection of calcification often assists in improving diagnostic accuracy
- Provides excellent visualization of extraocular muscles, orbital apex, and orbital vasculature

■ 2. Magnetic resonance imaging

- Indicated if CT is equivocal or if there is clinical suspicion of intracranial extension of an orbital abnormality, carotid–cavernous mass, or carotid–cavernous fistula

 Caveat: MRI is *contraindicated* if there is evidence or strong suspicion of metallic foreign bodies in or around the orbits.

Seizure Disorder (Epilepsy)

Presenting Signs and Symptoms

Sudden brief attacks of altered consciousness, motor activity, sensory phenomena, or inappropriate behavior

Common Causes

Congenital or developmental brain defects (usual onset of seizures at an early age)

Idiopathic (typically begins between ages 2 and 18)

Acute infection (febrile convulsion in child)

Trauma

Brain tumor

Metabolic disturbance (hypoglycemia, uremia, hepatic failure, electrolyte abnormality)

Cavernous malformation

Arteriovenous malformation

Toxic agent (lead, alcohol, cocaine)

Cerebral infarction or hemorrhage

Mesial temporal sclerosis

Approach to Diagnostic Imaging

Note: Neuroimaging is not recommended for a simple febrile seizure.

■ 1. Magnetic resonance imaging

- Most sensitive technique for detecting underlying cerebral abnormality (indicated in all adults with an unexplained first seizure)
- Follow-up MRI (at 3–6 months) is often of value if the initial examination failed to detect a source of the seizure disorder

Note: Examination consists of a routine brain study plus high-resolution, thin-section (2–3 mm) coronal T2-weighted images.

■ 2. Positron emission tomography

- Using F-18 deoxyglucose, this modality improves localization of the seizure focus, particularly in a patient with complex partial (temporal lobe), medically intractable seizures who has had a normal MRI scan
- Interictal hypometabolism

■ 3. Computed tomography

- Noncontrast scan is recommended as the initial study if the patient is in the immediate postictal state, or if residual neurologic deficit is present at the time of imaging (can detect important abnormalities, such as acute intracranial hemorrhage, that may require immediate medical or surgical treatment)
- Less sensitive than MRI

Note: In pediatric patients, contrast enhancement is generally not required because congenital anomalies, rather than tumor, are the most common structural cause of seizures.

Tinnitus

Presenting Signs and Symptoms

Perception of sound in the absence of an acoustic stimulus (ringing, buzzing, roaring, whistling, hissing) that may be intermittent, continuous, or pulsatile

Often associated with hearing loss

Common Causes

Virtually any ear disorder (obstruction, infection, cholesteatoma, neoplasm, eustachian tube obstruction, otosclerosis)

Cerebellopontine angle tumor

Drugs (salicylates, quinine, alcohol, certain antibiotics and diuretics)

Cardiovascular disease (hypertension, arteriosclerosis, aneurysm)

Trauma

Approach to Diagnostic Imaging

■ 1. Computed tomography (temporal bone)

- Preferred study for showing morphologic abnormality in the temporal bone

Note: Thin (1.5 mm) sections in axial and coronal planes are required.

■ 2. Magnetic resonance imaging

- If CT fails to detect a cause of symptoms, high-resolution, thin-section MRI is the preferred study for demonstrating small tumors (e.g., neurinoma) of the intracanalicular portion of the eighth cranial nerve as well as vascular abnormalities in the region of the cerebello-pontine angle
- Contrast infusion is often used, but may be unnecessary if thin-section (2–3 mm), axial, and coronal T1-weighted and coronal T2-weighted fast spin-echo images are obtained
- Thin-section MRI provides superb visualization of the inner ear structures and may be considered the initial study in the workup of tinnitus

Transient Ischemic Attacks

Presenting Sign and Symptom

Focal neurologic deficit that resolves fully within 24 h (sudden onset and brief duration)

Common Causes

Plaques or atherosclerotic ulcers involving the carotid or vertebral arteries in the neck

Emboli arising from mural thrombi in a diseased heart

Approach to Diagnostic Imaging

Note: The results of two clinical trials indicate the need to accurately detect carotid artery stenosis: (1) NASCET confirmed the value of carotid endarterectomy for stenosis (>70%) to prevent stroke and improve quality of life; (2) ACAST suggested surgery to prevent stroke for carotid stenosis (>60%).

■ 1. Duplex, color-flow Doppler ultrasound

- Accurate noninvasive screening study that combines high-resolution, real-time imaging of the carotid arteries with hemodynamic information about blood flow velocity provided by the Doppler technique
- Not needed if MR or CT angiography is performed

Note: Other noninvasive tests (ophthalmodyna-mometry, oculoplethysmography) are *not* indicated because they cannot accurately detect carotid plaques and ulcerations.

■ 2. Magnetic resonance angiography

- Accurate noninvasive screening study for detecting not only disease of the carotid bifurcation but also narrowing of the vertebral arteries
- Reconstitution sign (flow gap) confirms >60% stenosis (i.e., surgical disease).
- If surgery is contemplated, brain MR imaging and angiography can complete the diagnostic workup and preclude the need for catheter arteriography
- Contrast-enhanced MRA facilitates visualization of the aortic arch and the origins of the carotid and vertebral arteries

■ 3. Echocardiography

- Indicated to detect mural thrombi in the heart if no carotid lesion has been identified that could explain the patient's symptoms

■ 4. Computed tomography angiography

- Requires infusion of iodinated contrast material
- Diagnostic accuracy is similar to that of MRA for the detection of extra-axial and intra-axial arterial disease

Vertigo

Presenting Signs and Symptoms

Impression of movement in space or of objects, loss of
equilibrium, nausea, vomiting, nystagmus

Common Causes

Labyrinthine or middle ear infection or tumor
Head trauma
Toxic agent (alcohol, opiates, streptomycin)
Meniere's disease
Cerebellopontine angle tumor (neurinoma, meningioma,
metastasis, epidermoid)
Transient vertebrobasilar ischemic attacks
Motion sickness
Multiple sclerosis (focal brain stem lesion)

Approach to Diagnostic Imaging

■ 1. Magnetic resonance imaging

- Preferred study for detecting abnormalities of
the posterior fossa and cerebellopontine angle
(using high-resolution and thin-sections)
- Contrast enhancement is helpful for detecting a
small acoustic neurinoma

Note: If paramagnetic contrast material is not used,
an additional thin-section, coronal T2-weighted fast
spin-echo sequence should be obtained.

■ 2. Computed tomography

- Indicated if middle ear pathology is suspected

Note: Thin-section (1.5 mm) scanning in the axial and coronal planes using a bone-highlighting algorithm is required.

Unilateral Optic Nerve Impairment

Presenting Signs and Symptoms

Purely monocular visual loss

Normal ocular examination (or only optic atrophy) of both the symptomatic and asymptomatic eye

Common Causes

Optic neuritis (e.g., in association with multiple sclerosis)

Ischemic optic neuropathy

Compressive–infiltrative optic neuropathies (optic nerve glioma, lymphoma, leukemia, sarcoidosis)

Extrinsic compression by orbital mass (meningioma, metastasis, hemangioma, lymphangioma, dermoid, lymphoma)

Orbital pseudotumor

Thyroid ophthalmopathy

Approach to Diagnostic Imaging

■ 1. Computed tomography

- Axial 3-mm axial sections provide clear distinction of the optic nerves, extraocular muscles, and the globe, as well as calcification

- Because CT is superb for detecting the presence of calcification (very useful in the differential diagnosis of orbital masses) and orbital fat provides excellent contrast, some recommend this modality as the initial and often the definitive imaging study for orbital pathology.

■ 2. Magnetic resonance imaging

- Has the advantage of multiplanar imaging
- Very useful for delineating optic nerve pathology

> **Note:** Contrast enhancement and fat suppression generally are required to detect orbital masses.

Optic Chiasm Lesion

Presenting Signs and Symptoms

Bitemporal visual-field defects (although deficit may be substantially greater in one eye than in the other)

Common Causes

Pituitary tumor
Parasellar mass (meningioma, craniopharyngioma, aneurysm)
Multiple sclerosis
Sarcoidosis

Approach to Diagnostic Imaging

■ 1. Magnetic resonance imaging

- Preferred study for detecting a lesion compressing the optic chiasm because of its ability to image the sella and parasellar regions in the axial, coronal, and sagittal planes
- Can clearly demonstrate the entire course of the optic nerves, optic chiasm, and optic radiations, as well as the cavernous sinuses and carotid arteries

Note: Paramagnetic contrast enhancement is often helpful when multiple sclerosis or sarcoidosis is suspected.

Postchiasmal Visual System Dysfunction

Presenting Signs and Symptoms

Bilateral homonymous hemianopia (visual-field defects on same side of the vertical median for each eye)

Normal visual acuity, pupillary reflexes, and ophthalmoscopy

Common Causes

Tumor (primary or metastatic)
Abscess
Infarction
Arteriovenous malformation
Hematoma

Approach to Diagnostic Imaging

■ 1. Magnetic resonance imaging

- Preferred study for evaluating the optic tracts, optic radiations, and visual cortex

Brain Abscess

Presenting Signs and Symptoms

Headache
Nausea, vomiting
Papilledema
Lethargy
Seizures
Focal neurologic deficits
Fever, chills, and leukocytosis
Underlying immune deficiency

Common Causes

Direct extension of cranial infection (osteomyelitis, mastoiditis, sinusitis, subdural empyema)
Penetrating trauma
Hematogenous spread (bacterial endocarditis, intravenous drug abuse, bronchiectasis, congenital heart disease with right-to-left shunt)

Approach to Diagnostic Imaging

■ 1. Magnetic resonance imaging

- Most sensitive study for detecting the typically ring-enhancing mass lesion and associated edema and mass effect
- Superior to CT for detecting multiple brain abscesses
- Demonstrates restricted diffusion (increased signal on diffusion-weighted imaging)

■ 2. Computed tomography

- Contrast-enhanced study can identify the high-attenuation capsule surrounding the hypodense necrotic center (if MRI is not available)

Central Nervous System Manifestations in AIDS

Presenting Signs and Symptoms

Spectrum of neurologic deficits depending on region and extent of involvement

Common Causes

HIV encephalitis
Progressive multifocal leukoencephalopathy (PML)
Cytomegalovirus
Toxoplasmosis
Cryptococcosis
Lymphoma (primary CNS)

Approach to Diagnostic Imaging

■ 1. Magnetic resonance imaging

- Most sensitive imaging study in symptomatic patients for demonstrating single or multiple lesions of abnormal signal intensity or diffuse changes in the deep white matter
- If nonenhanced MRI is positive, contrast enhancement is helpful in differentiating abscess and lymphoma (enhancing) from HIV encephalitis and PML (nonenhancing)
- Elevated choline and lipid/lactate peaks on proton spectroscopy suggest lymphoma

HIV Encephalopathy

Presenting Signs and Symptoms

Progressive encephalopathy, somnolence, slow speech, word-finding difficulty, flat affect, and diminished attention in an HIV-positive patient

Approach to Diagnostic Imaging

■ 1. Magnetic resonance imaging

- In addition to showing central atrophy out of proportion to the patient's age, this modality is the most sensitive for demonstrating high-signal lesions (on T2-weighted images) that are focally or diffusely distributed throughout the deep white matter
- Demonstrates decreased signal intensity on T1-weighted images in the clivus and prominent lymphoid tonsillar tissue

---

Note: Although there is poor correlation between the extent of atrophy and the severity of dementia in AIDS, symptomatic HIV-positive patients are more than three times as likely to have abnormal MRI examinations. Routine MRI screening of neurologically asymptomatic HIV-positive patients is *not* cost-effective. When an abnormality is found on nonenhanced MRI, paramagnetic contrast material assists in distinguishing HIV encephalitis and PML (which do *not* enhance) from abscess and primary CNS lymphoma (which *do* enhance).

Acute Bacterial Meningitis

Presenting Signs and Symptoms

Prodromal respiratory illness, or sore throat, headache, stiff neck, fever, vomiting, seizures, impaired consciousness

Common Organisms

Meningococci, *Haemophilus influenzae* type b, pneumococci, gram-negative organisms

Common Causes

Extension from nearby infected structures (sinuses, mastoid air cells)

Communication of cerebrospinal fluid with exterior (penetrating trauma, myelomeningocele, spinal dermal sinus, neurosurgical procedures)

Approach to Diagnostic Imaging

Note: The most important role of imaging is to exclude a mass (abscess) prior to performance of a lumbar puncture (the primary diagnostic test).

▪ 1. Computed tomography (head)

- Contrast scans may demonstrate characteristic enhancement of the subarachnoid spaces, in addition to small ventricles and effacement of the sulci secondary to cerebral edema
- May demonstrate the underlying cause for the development of meningitis (brain abscess, sinus or mastoid infection, congenital anomaly)

Note: MRI may be normal in patients with meningitis if contrast material is not used.

Caveat: Because acute bacterial meningitis (especially meningococcal) can be rapidly lethal, use of antibiotics should *not* be delayed pending results of diagnostic tests.

Subacute/Chronic Meningitis

Presenting Signs and Symptoms

Similar to acute bacterial meningitis (but developing over weeks rather than days)

Common Causes

Chronic infection (fungal, tuberculosis, syphilis, amebic)
Immunosuppressive therapy
AIDS
Neoplasm (leukemia, lymphoma, melanoma, carcinomas, tumor seeding)
Sarcoidosis
Ruptured dermoid

Approach to Diagnostic Imaging

■ 1. Magnetic resonance imaging

- Contrast scans are required to demonstrate the characteristic enhancement of the subarachnoid spaces, as well as an underlying neoplasm
- Can demonstrate associated brain edema, abscess, or neoplasm, as well as inflammation of the paranasal sinuses or mastoids
- Superior to CT for evaluating complications of meningitis such as subdural empyema, dural venous thrombosis, infarction, and abscess

■ 2. Plain chest radiograph

- Indicated to search for evidence of underlying tuberculosis or sarcoidosis

Subdural Empyema

Presenting Signs and Symptoms

Headache
Lethargy
Vomiting
Fever
Focal neurologic deficits
Seizures
Often rapid clinical deterioration (an emergency condition)

Common Causes

Extension from nearby infected structure (sinusitis, ear infection, osteomyelitis, brain abscess)
Most common in children and young adult males because of the anatomic structure of the cribriform plate
Penetrating trauma
Surgical drainage of a subdural hematoma
Bacteremia (especially from pulmonary infection)

Approach to Diagnostic Imaging

■ 1. Computed tomography or magnetic resonance imaging

- Demonstrates characteristic crescentic or lentiform extra-axial fluid collection that is of low attenuation on CT and mildly hyperintense to CSF on T2-weighted MRI
- Contrast studies show an intensely enhancing surrounding membrane

Note: Subdural empyema is far easier to visualize using MRI (because it can be extremely difficult on CT to detect the extracerebral collection adjacent to the skull unless wider windowing is used).

Acoustic Neurinoma

Presenting Signs and Symptoms

Hearing loss (sensorineural)
Tinnitus
Dizziness and unsteadiness

Approach to Diagnostic Imaging

■ 1. Magnetic resonance imaging

- Preferred study for detecting abnormalities of the cerebellopontine angle and posterior fossa using thin-section axial and coronal T1- and T2-weighted images
- May identify small intracanalicular tumors because of their intense contrast enhancement

Note: A thin-section, multiplanar, high-resolution study is required.

■ 2. Computed tomography

- Indicated if there is conductive hearing loss to evaluate bony abnormality in the petrous portion of the temporal bone

Note: Thin sections with bone windows are required.

Brain Neoplasm

Presenting Signs and Symptoms

Slowly progressive focal neurologic deficits (depending on the site of the lesion)

Nonfocal symptoms due to increased intracranial pressure

Seizures

Cognitive symptoms (drowsiness, lethargy, personality changes, impaired mental faculties, psychotic episodes)

Signs of herniation

Approach to Diagnostic Imaging

■ 1. Magnetic resonance imaging

- Preferred screening technique for detecting and characterizing intracranial masses (may not require contrast infusion)
- Surgical planning or tumor biopsy can be performed using an MRI-compatible stereotaxic frame
- Potentially improved specificity using proton spectroscopy
- Functional MRI and Diffusion Tensor Tractography are often helpful in presurgical planning

---

Note: CT is only indicated to demonstrate bone erosion (especially at the skull base) and intra-mass calcification (although gradient-recalled echo sequences increase the sensitivity of MRI to mineralization), as well as for CT-guided biopsy.

Epidural Spinal Metastases

Presenting Signs and Symptoms

Back pain
Progressive weakness and sensory symptoms (numbness and paresthesias)
Bowel and bladder dysfunction
Corticospinal tract signs

Common Primary Neoplasms

Lung
Breast
Prostate
Melanoma
Lymphoma
Kidney
Gastrointestinal tract

Approach to Diagnostic Imaging

■ 1. Plain spinal radiograph

- Demonstrates single or multiple, lytic or blastic lesions or compression fractures in 60–85% of patients with epidural metastases
- Ineffective for detecting early metastases because about 50% of cancellous bone in the region must be destroyed before lytic lesions show on plain radiographs

■ 2. Magnetic resonance imaging

- Most sensitive technique that can simultaneously demonstrate the bone marrow abnormalities of vertebral metastases (hypointense on T1-weighted images and hyperintense on T2-weighted and STIR images) and epidural extension effacing and displacing the spinal cord and nerve roots

---

Note: Differentiation of benign from malignant causes of vertebral body fracture can be accomplished by MRI. Factors consistent with malignancy include complete (or nearly so) tumor replacement of marrow in vertebral bodies and posterior elements, sparing of disc spaces, multilevel involvement, and paravertebral masses.

 Caveat: Contrast enhancement may obscure evidence of destructive changes in the vertebral bodies. Always perform a nonenhanced T1-weighted sagittal image sequence before giving paramagnetic contrast material.

Intracerebral Metastases

Presenting Signs and Symptoms

Headache
Focal neurologic deficits
Drowsiness
Papilledema
Seizures

Common Primary Neoplasms

Lung
Breast
Melanoma
Gastrointestinal tract
Kidney
Thyroid

Approach to Diagnostic Imaging

■ 1. Magnetic resonance imaging

- Nonenhanced MRI is extremely sensitive for detecting brain metastases (predominantly located at the gray–white junction)
- Contrast enhancement makes this modality even more sensitive for detecting brain metastases
- Associated vasogenic edema, seen on T2-weighted images, consists of pure edema with no tumor extension

Note: Enhanced CT is limited by artifacts in the temporal lobes and posterior fossa.

Pineal Region Tumors

Presenting Signs and Symptoms

Precocious puberty (especially in boys)

Paralysis of upward gaze (Parinaud's syndrome relating to compression of tectal plate)

Noncommunicating obstructive hydrocephalus (due to obstruction at the aqueduct of Sylvius)

Papilledema and other signs of increased intracranial pressure

Common Causes

Germinoma

Teratoma

Glioma

Approach to Diagnostic Imaging

■ 1. Magnetic resonance imaging

- ■ Most sensitive study for detecting a neoplasm in the pineal region, but rarely specific enough to provide a histologic diagnosis (except for the heterogeneous appearance of intratumoral fat and calcium in a teratoma)

- ■ Combination of axial and sagittal images permits visualization of even small tumors. Obstruction of the aqueduct may obliterate the normal pulsatile signal void

- ■ A benign pineal cyst may measure up to 25 mm and have a signal intensity not precisely the same as that of cerebrospinal fluid. The benign nature of the lesion is confirmed by the absence of obstructive hydrocephalus and the unchanging size on serial examinations

 Caveat: Enhancement may occur normally in the pineal region. This appearance should *not* be mistaken for tumor enhancement.

Acute Brain Infarction (Stroke)

Presenting Signs and Symptoms

Abrupt, dramatic onset of focal neurologic deficit that
does not resolve within 24 h

Possible headache or seizure

Common Causes

Infarction (secondary to an embolism from the heart or
extracranial circulation or to hemorrhage)

Narrowing of intracranial or extracranial artery (atherosclerosis, thrombus, dissection, vasculitis)

Thrombus of the cerebral venous system

Rupture of an aneurysm or arteriovenous malformation
(causing subarachnoid hemorrhage or intracerebral
hematoma)

Decreased perfusion pressure or increased blood viscos-
ity with inadequate blood flow reaching the brain

Hypertension, coagulopathy, or amyloid angiopathy
causing intracerebral hematoma

Approach to Diagnostic Imaging

■ 1. Computed tomography (noncontrast ± contrast)

- Preferred initial procedure for assessing a suspected
  acute stroke because it can:
    - Rule out hemorrhage (subarachnoid or intrace-
      rebral)
    - Define patterns of early ischemic injury (blurred
      putamen, effaced sulci, dense middle cerebral
      artery)
    - Show areas of abnormal vascular calcification
      (e.g., giant aneurysm)
    - Exclude a mass lesion
- CT angiography delineates vascular occlusion or
  aneurysm

- CT perfusion (CBF, CBV, transit time, TTP) after rapid-bolus iodinated contrast material can better detect a hypoperfused abnormality to potentially distinguish irreversible infarction from surrounding salvageable ischemic penumbra

---

Note: The above information is critical for the clinician faced with determining the need for lumbar puncture, vascular surgery, anticoagulation, and thrombolytic therapy.

■ 2. Magnetic resonance imaging

- The combination of nonenhanced MR imaging and MR angiography is more sensitive than CT for detecting infarction and ischemic edema (especially involving the brainstem), clearly delineating an occluded or stenotic artery or vein, and distinguishing hemorrhagic from ischemic infarction

 Caveat: Arteriography is indicated *only* if noninvasive studies suggest an underlying aneurysm, AVM, or vascular occlusion *and* a surgical or interventional radiologic procedure is seriously being considered.

■ 3. Diffusion-weighted magnetic resonance imaging

- This most sensitive marker of acute infarction is generally positive within 2 h of the clinical event and thus plays a critical diagnostic role
- The hyperintense signal (hypointensity on ADC map) is possibly related to cytotoxic (intracellular) edema
- A negative study is highly predictive for excluding an acute brain infarction and thus is valuable in directing further diagnostic and therapeutic planning
- Combination MR perfusion study with diffusion may predict ischemic penumbra (tissue at risk) and need for emergent clot lysis therapy.

Intraparenchymal Cerebral Hemorrhage

Presenting Signs and Symptoms

Abrupt onset of headache followed by steadily increasing
neurologic deficits
Loss of consciousness
Nausea, vomiting
Delirium
Focal or generalized seizures
Signs of transtentorial herniation

Common Causes

Trauma
Hypertensive hematoma (common locations: putamen-
external capsule, caudate, thalamus, pons, cerebellum,
cerebral hemisphere)
Congenital aneurysm or arteriovenous malformation
Amyloid angiopathy (causes polar hemorrhage)
Mycotic aneurysm
Blood dyscrasia (bleeding diathesis)
Collagen disease
Hemorrhagic infarction (arterial or venous)
Metastases (e.g., melanoma)
Glioblastoma multiforme
Cavernous malformations

Approach to Diagnostic Imaging

■ 1. Computed tomography

- Preferred imaging technique for detecting a focal region of increased attenuation within the brain parenchyma in *acute* trauma, suspected aneurysm rupture (because of superior detection of subarachnoid hemorrhage and patient comfort), or hypertensive episode
- CT angiography can detect aneurysm or vascular occlusion

 Caveat: Although it is unusual, CT may at times fail to detect subarachnoid blood found at lumbar puncture.

■ 2. Magnetic resonance imaging

- Preferred study for detecting *subacute* and *chronic* stages of intraparenchymal hemorrhage
- An *acute* hematoma (intracellular deoxyhemoglobin) appears hypointense on T2-weighted images; a *subacute* hematoma (methemoglobin) is hyperintense on T1-weighted images
- Hemosiderin- or ferritin-laden macrophages that develop due to prior bleeding appear as hypointense foci on T2-weighted images, persist throughout the patient's life, and are best seen on gradient echo images
- MR angiography or venography may prove helpful for detecting aneurysms, arteriovenous malformations, or venous occlusions

■ 3. Arteriography

- Remains the "gold standard" for imaging suspected aneurysms or arteriovenous malformations and also provides a therapeutic portal
- Best modality for visualizing narrowing of branch vessels due to arteritis

Subarachnoid Hemorrhage

Presenting Signs and Symptoms

Sudden onset of excruciating headache

Rapid loss of consciousness

Vomiting

Severe neck stiffness (usually not present initially but occurring within 24h)

Progressive palsies (reflecting pressure effects on the third, fourth, fifth, and sixth cranial nerves)

Common Causes

Trauma

Rupture of congenital intracranial aneurysm

Arteriovenous malformation

Mycotic aneurysm (in patients who have infective endocarditis or systemic infection or are immuno-compromised)

Blood dyscrasia (bleeding diathesis)

Approach to Diagnostic Imaging

■ 1. Computed tomography

- Preferred study for demonstrating acute sub-arachnoid hemorrhage
- Initial noncontrast scan to detect the presence of high-density blood in the subarachnoid space
- Subsequent contrast-enhanced CT angiography may detect the underlying aneurysm or vascular malformation

 Caveat: Lumbar puncture to demonstrate blood in the subarachnoid space is indicated *only* if CT fails to make the diagnosis *and* shows no evidence of a mass or obstructive hydrocephalus (lest herniation occur).

■ 2. Arteriography

- Indicated to localize and characterize the anatomy of an aneurysm or arteriovenous malformation and for neurointerventional therapy
- If there is an aneurysm, must also evaluate for vasospasm

Note: Must selectively catheterize both carotid and one vertebral artery (if reflux into the other).

■ 3. Magnetic resonance imaging

- Can detect subarachnoid hemorrhage in the acute stage using FLAIR pulse sequences
- Superior to CT for demonstrating chronic blood staining of the meninges (hemosiderosis)
- Role of MRA in aneurysm detection is emerging, although the "gold standard" remains selective catheter arteriography

Cerebral Aneurysm

Presenting Signs and Symptoms

Asymptomatic

Signs of intraparenchymal or subarachnoid hemorrhage (if rupture)

Compression of cranial nerves or brain parenchyma (if large)

Common Causes

Congenital (berry aneurysm)

Atherosclerotic (often giant)

Mycotic

Trauma

Association with large AVMs

Approach to Diagnostic Imaging

■ 1. Computed tomography

- Detects subarachnoid hemorrhage and intracerebral hematoma in the acute setting
- CT angiography delineates aneurysms of the circle of Willis

■ 2. Arteriography

- If cerebral aneurysm is suggested by CT or MRI evidence of intraparenchymal or subarachnoid hemorrhage, arteriography can:
  - Identify the presence of any and all aneurysms
  - Delineate the relationship of a given aneurysm to the parent vessel and adjacent penetrating branches
  - Define the potential for collateral circulation to the brain
  - Assess for vasospasm
  - Act as the portal for neurointerventional therapy (e.g., ballooning)

■ 3. Computed tomography or magnetic resonance imaging

- Can demonstrate a patent suprasellar aneurysm as an intensely enhancing mass (CT) or as a high-velocity flow void with signal heterogeneity due to turbulence (MRI)

■ 4. MR or CT angiography

- Demonstrates the parent artery and the size and orientation of the neck and dome of the aneurysm
- Useful screening study in asymptomatic patients, as well as in those with a family history of aneurysms or a familial disorder associated with cerebral aneurysms

---

Note: Future technical refinements will permit detection of progressively smaller aneurysms.

Arteriovenous Malformation

Presenting Signs and Symptoms

Asymptomatic

Sudden headache and neurologic deficits (secondary to intraparenchymal or subarachnoid hemorrhage)

Focal seizures (incited by the lesion)

Progressive focal neurologic sensorimotor deficit (due to enlarging arteriovenous malformation acting as a mass or progressive ischemic lesion)

May have arterial bruit detectable on the overlying cranial vault

Better prognosis than berry aneurysm rupture

Common Cause

Congenital tangle of dilated blood vessels with direct flow from arterial afferents into venous efferents

Approach to Diagnostic Imaging

■ 1. Magnetic resonance imaging

- Demonstrates AVMs as tangled flow voids with prominent feeding and draining vessels

- Superior to CT for demonstrating *subacute* and *chronic* hemorrhage and secondary changes (mass effect, edema), as well as ischemic changes in the adjacent brain

- Optimal for detecting low-flow and angiographically occult vascular malformations (cavernous angioma, telangiectasia, venous angioma)

■ 2. Arteriography

- Required to precisely demonstrate the anatomic blood supply and drainage prior to any surgical or neurointerventional procedure
- Can distinguish among pial, dural, and mixed types of AVMs

Lacunar Infarction

Presenting Sign and Symptom

Focal neurologic deficit that can be pinpointed to a locus less than 15 mm in diameter

Common Causes

Embolic, atherosclerotic, or thrombotic lesions in long, single, penetrating end-arterioles (or the parent vessel from which these perforators emerge) supplying the deep cerebral white matter, thalamus, basal ganglia-capsular region, and pons

Hypertension (common)

Approach to Diagnostic Imaging

■ 1. Magnetic resonance imaging

- *Only* modality that can consistently demonstrate the well-delineated round or slit-like lesions that are hypointense to brain on T1-weighted images and hyperintense to brain on intermediate and T2-weighted images
- Hypointensity on T2-weighted and gradient echo images denotes chronic blood products

- Diffusion-weighted imaging is extremely helpful in distinguishing acute(hyperintense on race map) from chronic lacunes

Note: Because of their small size, most true lacunar infarctions are difficult to see on CT scans.

- MR or CT angiography is usually negative because of the involvement of small blood vessels (arterioles), but it can detect occlusion of a parent artery (e.g., middle cerebral artery occlusion causing infarction in the distribution of the lenticulostriate perforators) when the lacunar distribution of the infarction is larger than expected.

Acute Head Trauma

Presenting Signs and Symptoms

Focal neurologic deficits (caused by intracerebral and extracerebral hematomas)

Generalized or focal cerebral edema that may lead to symptoms of herniation (through tentorium or foramen magnum)

Concussion (post-traumatic loss of consciousness)

Approach to Diagnostic Imaging

■ 1. Computed tomography

- Preferred study for detecting skull fracture, *acute* intraparenchymal bleeding, and extra-axial hemorrhage (acute subdural and epidural hematoma)

- The use of wider windows improves ability of CT images to delineate isodense extracerebral hematoma

- Demonstrates ventricular shift and sulcal effacement, subtle findings that should raise suspicion of an isodense subdural hematoma

■ 2. Magnetic resonance imaging

- Indicated only in those unusual acute cases in which CT has failed to detect an abnormality in the presence of strong clinical suspicion of intracranial hemorrhage (primarily in the posterior fossa, temporal and inferior frontal lobes, or high on the convexity, areas in which CT may be limited because of overlying bone)

- Particularly valuable in *subacute* and *chronic* phases of head trauma to define temporal and inferior frontal lobe hemorrhagic contusion and edema, as well as shear injuries (subtle hemorrhage seen as low signal on gradient echo images) at the gray–white junctions and posterior corpus callosum

Note: There is *no* indication for plain skull radiography in this condition. The mere detection of a skull fracture generally has little effect on subsequent medical or surgical management. In addition, skull fractures usually are easily recognizable on CT, which can also delineate any accompanying abnormality in the underlying brain.

Epidural Hematoma

Presenting Signs and Symptoms

Symptoms developing within minutes or hours after injury (often after a lucid interval of relative neurologic normalcy)

Increasing headache, deterioration of consciousness, motor dysfunction, and pupillary changes indicate an *emergency* situation

Common Cause

Trauma (causing arterial laceration in the epidural space)

Approach to Diagnostic Imaging

■ 1. Computed tomography

- Preferred study for demonstrating the characteristic appearance of a collection that is hyperintense hemorrhage convex to the brain that is located in the temporal region (middle meningeal artery) and often associated with a skull fracture

Note: There is *no* indication for plain skull radiographs in this condition.

Acute Subdural Hematoma

Presenting Signs and Symptoms

Progressive neurologic deterioration with signs of herniation
Progressive loss of consciousness
Hemiplegia

Common Cause

Head trauma

Approach to Diagnostic Imaging

■ 1. Computed tomography

- Preferred study for detecting the characteristically hyperintense, medially concave, lenticular extra-axial collection of blood in the subdural space

 Caveat: Thin subdural hematomas may be obscured by overlying bone (especially if they are located high on the convexity). Subfrontal or subtemporal hematomas may be difficult to detect on axial views and may require coronal reformatting or direct coronal imaging.

- Effacement of cortical sulci on three or more adjacent images
- Hematoma may be isodense if the hematocrit is less than 30 mL/dL

■ 2. Magnetic resonance imaging

- Not as specific for detecting acute bleeding, but ability of MRI to directly obtain coronal images may be of value if CT fails to demonstrate a subdural hematoma in the face of strongly suggestive clinical findings

---

Note: There is *no* indication for plain skull films in this clinical setting.

Chronic Subdural Hematoma

Presenting Signs and Symptoms

History of head trauma (2–4 weeks or more prior to clinical presentation) that may have been relatively trivial and forgotten

Increasing headache

Fluctuating drowsiness or confusion

Mild-to-moderate hemiparesis

Typically occurs in alcoholics and patients older than age 50

Common Cause

Head trauma

Approach to Diagnostic Imaging

■ 1. Magnetic resonance imaging

- Preferred study for detecting hemorrhages more than a few days old as extracerebral lesions on both T1- and T2-weighted sequences
- Of particular value in detecting hemorrhages in the posterior fossa and high on the convexity (difficult areas for CT because of bone artifacts)

- Clearly defines secondary findings (brain contusion or hematoma, axonal shear injury at the gray–white junction and posterior corpus callosum, occipital infarction secondary to prior transtentorial herniation, communicating hydrocephalus, atrophy)
- Subtle axonal shear injuries may only be detected on gradient echo pulse sequences

Note: Unlike CT, where hemorrhage becomes isodense after several weeks and thus may be impossible to recognize, hemorrhage on MRI remains hypointense for the lifetime of the patient.

Cervical Spine Trauma

Approach to Diagnostic Imaging

Note: According to the NEXUS trial, imaging of the cervical spine is not necessary if all five of these criteria are met:
  Absence of posterior midline tenderness
  Absence of focal neurologic deficit
  Normal level of alertness
  No evidence of intoxication
  Absence of painful distracting injury

■ 1. Plain skeletal radiograph

- Preferred initial screening procedure that is quickly and inexpensively performed without significant disruption of other resuscitation efforts

Note: Cross-table lateral view is generally obtained first, to avoid moving a patient who might have a cervical fracture; if it appears normal, additional films (including odontoid, oblique, flexion, and extension views) may be obtained.

 Caveat: It is absolutely *imperative* that all seven cervical vertebral bodies be seen, to avoid missing a lower cervical spine fracture obscured by the shoulders. If the entire cervical spine is not seen, the film must be repeated with the shoulders lowered.

■ 2. Computed tomography

- Indicated if plain skeletal radiographs are equivocal, fail to adequately image portions of the spine, or show a complex fracture of the cervical spine (especially involving the foramen transversarium housing the vertebral artery, which may be compromised by cervical trauma)
- May be required in a trauma victim whose plain films are negative but who has substantial neck pain or neurologic deficits

Note: Cervical spine CT is cost-effective and may actually be cost-saving in patients with a high probability of fracture (especially if they are already scheduled to undergo head CT) because of the decreased number of second imaging examinations resulting from frequently inadequate radiographic studies and in view of the high cost in dollars and health for the rare fracture missed from radiography that leads to severe neurologic deficit. Radiography remains the most cost-effective imaging option in patients with a low probability of injury.

■ 3. Magnetic resonance imaging

- Best procedure for detecting cord contusion and edema (and its sequela, myelomalacia), herniated disk, canal compromise, or epidural hematoma complicating trauma to the cervical spine

Note: In a patient with suspected nerve root avulsion, either CT myelography or MRI can confirm the diagnosis.

Blow-Out Fracture of the Orbit

Presenting Signs and Symptoms

History of trauma
Extraocular eye movement abnormality

Approach to Diagnostic Imaging

■ 1. Plain radiograph (Waters view)

- Most cost-effective screening study for showing bony discontinuity and the presence of a soft-tissue mass in the superior aspect of the maxillary antrum

■ 2. Computed tomography (axial and coronal)

- Definitive studies for showing the fracture and the extent of herniation of orbital tissues through the defect into the superior aspect of the maxillary antrum

---

Note: If a blow-out fracture is suspected clinically, CT can be the initial imaging procedure (omitting plain radiography).

Facial Fracture

Presenting Signs and Symptoms

Facial swelling and ecchymoses

Approach to Diagnostic Imaging

■ 1. Plain radiograph

- Preferred screening study for demonstrating facial fractures (most commonly involving the nose, zygomatic arches, lateral walls of the maxillary antra, and floors of the orbits)

■ 2. Computed tomography

- Indicated if plain radiographs demonstrate a complex fracture that must be defined or suggest a blow-out fracture of the floor of the orbit, and when there is a strong clinical suspicion of fracture and a plain radiograph may not be needed

Note: Both axial *and* coronal 3-mm-section scans are usually required for full evaluation.

Temporal Bone Fracture

Presenting Signs and Symptoms

Various symptoms depending on the fracture site (hearing loss, vertigo, nystagmus, facial paralysis)
Hemorrhage behind the tympanic membrane

Common Cause

Trauma

Approach to Diagnostic Imaging

■ 1. Computed tomography

- In addition to demonstrating the lucent fracture line (often requiring thin cuts), CT may show secondary signs of fracture such as fluid within the mastoid air cells or tympanic cavity, intracranial gas, gas within the temporomandibular joint, and disruption of the ossicular chain

Note: Always check the temporomandibular fossa for dislocation.

Acromegaly/Gigantism

Presenting Signs and Symptoms

Soft-tissue and bony overgrowth (increased size of hands, feet, jaw, and cranium)

Coarsening of facial features

Peripheral neuropathies

Headache

Impaired glucose tolerance

Common Cause

Pituitary adenoma (excessive secretion of growth hormone)

Approach to Diagnostic Imaging

■ 1. Magnetic resonance imaging

- Preferred study for detecting and defining the extent of the underlying pituitary tumor (superb sensitivity and multiplanar capability)
- Thin-section coronal and sagittal T1-weighted images and coronal T2-weighted images should be obtained
- Paramagnetic contrast material is generally not required for initial screening
- Permits clear distinction of the sphenoid sinus and the position of the carotid artery for surgical planning
- If an aneurysm is suspected on MR imaging, MR angiography is obtained

Note: There is *no* indication for plain radiographs of the sella in this condition.

Diabetes Insipidus

Presenting Signs and Symptoms

Excretion of excessive quantities of urine (polyuria) that is very dilute but otherwise normal

Excessive thirst (polydipsia)

Dehydration and hypovolemia (develops rapidly if urinary losses are not continuously replaced)

Common Causes

PRIMARY (IDIOPATHIC)

Marked decrease in hypothalamic nuclei of neuro-hypophyseal system and deficient production of vasopressin (antidiuretic hormone)

SECONDARY (ACQUIRED)

Hypophysectomy

Cranial injury (especially basal skull fracture)

Suprasellar and intrasellar neoplasm (primary or metastatic)

Histiocytosis X

Granulomatous disease (tuberculosis, sarcoidosis)

Vascular lesion (aneurysm, thrombosis)

Infection (encephalitis, meningitis)

Approach to Diagnostic Imaging

■ 1. Magnetic resonance imaging

- Preferred study for demonstrating any underlying lesion of the hypothalamus, pituitary gland, or pituitary stalk (superb sensitivity, multiplanar capability)

Note: High-resolution, thin-section study is required; contrast enhancement improves sensitivity.

Galactorrhea/Amenorrhea

Presenting Signs and Symptoms

WOMEN

Galactorrhea
Menstrual disturbances
Infertility
Symptoms of estrogen deficiency (hot flashes, dyspareunia)

MEN

Loss of libido and potency
Infertility (occasional galactorrhea or gynecomastia)

Common Causes

Prolactinoma of pituitary gland
Drugs (phenothiazines, antihypertensives)
Primary hypothyroidism
Hypothalamic/pituitary stalk disease

Approach to Diagnostic Imaging

■ 1. Magnetic resonance imaging

- Preferred study for demonstrating the prolactin-secreting pituitary microadenoma (usually <1 cm) that is the underlying cause in about 50% of patients
- Requires thin-section imaging in both coronal and sagittal planes

Note: There is *no* indication for plain films of the sella in this condition.

Hypopituitarism

Presenting Signs and Symptoms

Variable depending on which specific pituitary hormones are deficient (gonadotropins, growth hormone, thyroid-stimulating hormone, adrenocorticotropic hormone)

Common Causes

PITUITARY LESION

Tumor (adenoma, craniopharyngioma)
Infarction or ischemic necrosis
Inflammatory or infiltrative process (e.g., sarcoidosis)
Iatrogenic (irradiation or surgical removal)

HYPOTHALAMIC LESION

Tumor
Inflammation
Trauma

Approach to Diagnostic Imaging

■ 1. Magnetic resonance imaging

- Preferred study because of its superb sensitivity and ability to directly image the sella and para-sellar regions in multiple planes

> **Note:** Paramagnetic contrast enhancement is helpful in older patients with Addison's disease and in detecting sarcoidosis. To define tiny microadenomas, imaging should begin immediately after contrast infusion to avoid obscuring a late-enhancing adenoma.
>
> There is *no* indication for plain films of the sella in this condition.

Cauda Equina Syndrome

Presenting Signs and Symptoms

Bilateral radiculopathy
Saddle anesthesia
Flaccid paralysis
Urinary retention

Causes

Ruptured intervertebral disk
Tumor
Infection
Trauma

Approach to Diagnostic Imaging

■ 1. Magnetic resonance imaging

- Preferred study for demonstrating complete subarachnoid block and the underlying cause
- Imaging in the sagittal and axial planes is required
  from the conus to the bottom of the thecal sac

Note: This is a surgical emergency requiring immediate imaging for a precise diagnosis.

Herniated Nucleus Pulposus

Presenting Signs and Symptoms

Pain in the distribution of compressed nerve roots (may be sudden and severe or more insidious)

Pain increased by movement or Valsalva maneuver

Paresthesias or numbness in the sensory distribution of the affected roots

Reduced or absent deep tendon reflexes in the distribution of involved nerve roots

Weakness and eventual atrophy of muscles supplied by affected nerves

Positive straight leg raising test (lumbosacral region)

Urinary incontinence or retention (from loss of sphincter function in lumbosacral involvement)

Most common in the lower lumbosacral and lower cervical regions

Common Cause

Degenerative disk disease

Approach to Diagnostic Imaging

■ 1. Magnetic resonance imaging

- Most sensitive study for demonstrating bulging, protrusion, extrusion, or free fragmentation of disk material, as well as impingement on the conus and individual spinal nerve roots
- Can show degeneration of the disk as loss of signal on T2-weighted images (although this may be of little clinical importance)
- Can distinguish among canal stenosis, degenerative facet overgrowth, herniated disk, and synovial cyst
- Permits routine visualization of conus medullaris

■ 2. Computed tomography

- Useful for detecting herniated disk and canal stenosis, but limited by contrast resolution, single imaging plane, poor visualization of the conus without intrathecal contrast material, and poor assessment of the postoperative spine. Excellent for bone anatomy.

 Caveat: *Plain spinal radiographs* may demonstrate disk space narrowing and hypertrophic spurring. However, they do not show whether there is critical impingement on the vertebral canal or nerve roots, and are therefore of little value when MRI or CT is employed. *Myelography* should be reserved for special applications, often related to surgical planning.

Sciatica

Presenting Signs and Symptoms

Pain radiating down one or both buttocks and the posterior aspect of the leg(s) to below the knee (the distribution of the sciatic nerve)

Common Causes

Peripheral nerve root compression (intervertebral disk protrusion or intraspinal tumor)

Compression within the spinal canal or intervertebral foramen (tumor, osteoarthritis, spondylolisthesis)

Approach to Diagnostic Imaging

■ 1. Magnetic resonance imaging

- Most sensitive study for demonstrating bulging, protrusion, extrusion, or free fragmentation of disk material, as well as impingement on the spinal cord, conus, and individual nerve roots

■ 2. Computed tomography

- Still valuable for detecting herniated disk and bony foraminal or canal stenosis
- Disadvantages include poor visualization of the conus, inability to distinguish herniated disk from scar in the postoperative spine, essentially single axial-plane imaging, and radiation exposure

 Caveat: *Plain spinal radiographs* may demonstrate disk space narrowing and hypertrophic spurring. However, they do not show whether there is critical impingement on the spinal cord or nerve roots. *Myelography* is not indicated in the evaluation of sciatica and generally is not required if MRI or CT has been performed.

Scoliosis

Presenting Signs and Symptoms

Structural lateral curvature of the spine that may be suspected when one shoulder appears higher than the other or if clothes do not hang straight

Fatigue in the lumbar region after prolonged sitting or standing that may be associated with muscular backaches

Common Causes

Idiopathic

Vertebral anomaly

Hydromyelia and dysraphic states

Approach to Diagnostic Imaging

■ 1. Plain spinal radiograph

- Demonstrates the site and severity of the curvature (typically convex to the right in the thoracic area and to the left in the lumbar area so that the right shoulder is higher than the left)

■ 2. Magnetic resonance imaging

- Indicated to exclude an intraspinal abnormality if scoliosis is severe or has an early age of onset, or if plain radiographs show a vertebral anomaly
- The cervicomedullary junction should be reviewed to detect low-lying cerebellar tissue

---

Note: MRI is required to detect serious anomalies, such as tethered cord, that must be addressed before the spine undergoes mechanical straightening. Coverage from the cervicomedullary junction to the sacral level is generally needed (T1-weighted images are often sufficient).

Spinal Stenosis

Presenting Signs and Symptoms

Pain (and at times cramping) in the buttocks, thighs, or calves on walking, running, or climbing stairs, not relieved by standing still but by flexing the back, sitting, or lying down

Common Causes

Degenerative disease (hypertrophy of facets or ligamentum flavum, disk protrusion, postoperative scarring, synovial cyst)
Paget's disease
Achondroplasia
Trauma
Severe spondylolisthesis

Approach to Diagnostic Imaging

■ 1. Magnetic resonance imaging or computed tomography

- Demonstrate bony and soft-tissue changes causing compression of the thecal sac or spinal cord centrally, as well as encroachment on the nerve root in the neural foramen or lateral recess

- MRI is the study of choice because of multiplanar capability and ability to better visualize the conus, while CT is superior for demonstrating bony degenerative changes
- Associated herniated disk may occur, but not at the level of the spondylolisthesis

 Caveat: *Plain spinal radiographs* may demonstrate disk space narrowing and hypertrophic spurring. However, they do not show whether there is critical impingement on the spinal cord or nerve roots. Disk space narrowing and vertebral body alignment are better defined using MRI. *Myelography* is not indicated (except in some cases for presurgical planning) to evaluate disease involving the intervertebral disks or the spinal canal. Risk of epidural injection and severe discomfort are greatest in patients with spinal stenosis.

Failed Back Syndrome

Presenting Signs and Symptoms

No relief of neurologic symptoms after surgical procedure for herniated nucleus pulposus

Occurs in the lumbar region in about 10–25% of patients

Common Causes

Recurrent or residual disk

Scarring

Lateral or central canal stenosis

Adhesive arachnoiditis

Conus abnormality

Approach to Diagnostic Imaging

■ 1. Magnetic resonance imaging

- Most accurate technique for making the crucial distinction between recurrent/residual disk and scar

- Scar is usually hyperintense to the annulus on T2-weighted scans (recurrent disk is hypointense) and enhances homogeneously after contrast administration (chronic disk herniation may have some peripheral enhancement because of surrounding granulation tissue)

- Must be analyzed carefully for canal stenosis, far-lateral herniated disc, and conus mass

Syringomyelia/Hydromyelia

Presenting Signs and Symptoms

Spasticity and weakness of the lower extremities

Sensory defect (typically beginning in the cervical region and often extending to a cape-like defect over the shoulders and back)

Common Causes

Congenital (often associated with Chiari malformation and encephalocele)

Intramedullary tumor (if there is no associated Chiari I malformation)

Trauma (post-traumatic syrinx cystic myelomalacia)

Approach to Diagnostic Imaging

■ 1. Magnetic resonance imaging

- Demonstrates an atrophic (chronic) or enlarged spinal cord with central cystic, haustrated cavity
- Commonly associated with Chiari I malformation
- Upper margin of the hydromyelia cavity is at the level of the pyramidal decussation (cephalad cervical cord)
- If there is no Chiari malformation or the cystic central cord lesion does not respect the pyramidal decussation boundary and extends above the cervicomedullary junction, contrast infusion is indicated to detect an underlying spinal cord neoplasm (hemangioblastoma, ependymoma, astrocytoma)

Tethered Cord (Low Conus)

Presenting Signs and Symptoms

Low back pain
Dysesthesias
Neurogenic bladder
Spasticity
Congenital/developmental kyphoscoliosis

Approach to Diagnostic Imaging

■ 1. Magnetic resonance imaging

- Preferred study for showing the low-lying (below L2-L3 level), posteriorly tethered conus medullaris and thickened filum terminale that may terminate in a lipoma or dermoid

---

Note: MRI of the entire spine is generally performed to evaluate for hydrosyringomyelia and any abnormality at the cervicomedullary junction.

Transverse Myelitis (Acute)

Presenting Signs and Symptoms

Sudden onset of local back pain followed by sensory symptoms and motor weakness ascending from the feet

Urinary retention and loss of bowel control

Common Causes

Unknown (may be related to a prior viral illness, vasculitis, intravenous use of heroin or amphetamine, multiple sclerosis, AIDS myelopathy, or dural vascular malformation)

Approach to Diagnostic Imaging

■ 1. Magnetic resonance imaging

- Shows focal enlargement of the spinal cord
- T2-weighted imaging demonstrates high signal throughout the region of involvement
- Contrast enhancement suggests an acute or early subacute demyelinating abnormality
- Often assists in defining the etiology of a lesion by the distribution of hyperintense signal, best defined on axial T2-weighted images

---

Note: The role of MRI is more to exclude treatable conditions, such as unsuspected cord compression, than to make a specific diagnosis.

Anosmia

Presenting Sign and Symptom

Loss of sense of smell

Common Causes

Head trauma (especially in young adults)
Viral infection (especially in older adults)
Chronic nasal obstruction (polyps)
Neoplasm (interfering with olfactory apparatus)
Granulomatous disease
Male hypogonadism (Kallmann's syndrome)

Approach to Diagnostic Imaging

■ 1. Magnetic resonance imaging

- Can detect a subfrontal mass (e.g., meningioma, metastasis or direct extension from squamous cell carcinoma, esthesioneuroblastoma)
- Used for planning prior to surgery or radiation therapy

■ 2. Computed tomography

- Can detect a neoplasm or unsuspected fracture of the floor of the anterior cranial fossa
- Can demonstrate polyps or other neoplastic or granulomatous processes resulting in nasal obstruction

Bell's Palsy

Presenting Signs and Symptoms

Unilateral facial paralysis (sudden onset)
Pain behind the ear (may precede facial weakness)
Widening of palpebral fissure (prevents closure of eye)

Common Causes

Unknown (presumably swelling of the facial nerve due
to immune or viral disease with resultant ischemia
and compression of the nerve as it passes through its
narrow canal in the temporal bone)
Trauma, schwannoma, vascular malformation, sarcoidosis

Approach to Diagnostic Imaging

■ 1. Magnetic resonance imaging

- Indicated to exclude a mass or demyelinating lesion
within or adjacent to the facial nerve (from its brain
stem origin to the parotid gland) if symptoms are
recurrent, prolonged, progressive, or associated
with dysfunction of other cranial nerves

Note: High-resolution axial and coronal imaging
with contrast enhancement is required.

- Demonstrates contrast enhancement in almost
80% of patients with clinical Bell's palsy (most
commonly in the labyrinthine segment and
descending facial nerve canal) that may persist
past the point of clinical improvement

 Caveat: Unfortunately, the side of enhancement may not always correlate with the clinical
symptoms.

Cerebrospinal Fluid Leak

Presenting Signs and Symptoms

Leakage of CSF (identified by its glucose content) from the nose (rhinorrhea) or ears (otorrhea)

Common Causes

Fracture with dural tear

Communication develops between the subarachnoid space and the paranasal sinuses or the middle ear (in association with disruption of the tympanic membrane)

Approach to Diagnostic Imaging

■ 1. Radionuclide cisternography

- Procedure of choice that is extremely sensitive in demonstrating tiny amounts of radionuclide in cotton pledgets placed in the nostrils or the external ears

 Caveat: This technique is unsatisfactory for localizing the precise site of leakage.

■ 2. Computed tomography (CT cisternography)

- Thin-section scanning is performed both before and after the intrathecal injection of nonionic, iodinated contrast material via lumbar puncture

Note: Delayed imaging may be required a few hours later to detect subtle leakage.

 Caveat: CSF leakage often cannot be detected even using both radionuclide and CT cisternography.

■ 3. Magnetic resonance imaging

- Very high-resolution, thin-section, multiplanar T2-weighted imaging may detect the site of the leak

Multiple Sclerosis

Presenting Signs and Symptoms

Various focal neurologic dysfunctions characterized by
erratic remissions and exacerbations
Paresthesias (extremity, trunk, or face)
Weakness or clumsiness of leg or hand
Visual disturbances (optic neuritis)
Abnormalities of gait and coordination

Common Causes

Unknown (possibly viral or immune-related)
Increased risk in persons living in northern climates
(e.g., northern United States, Canada, Scandinavia)
before puberty

Approach to Diagnostic Imaging

■ 1. Magnetic resonance imaging

- Most sensitive study for detecting the scattered plaques of demyelination that are hyperintense to brain on T2-weighted sequences
- Greater specificity with lesions involving the inferior corpus callosum, peritemporal horn white matter, optic nerves or chiasm, and middle cerebral peduncle, as well as discrete lesions in the pons or the posterior column of the cervical portion of the spinal cord

---

Note: Lesions involving the optic nerve or chiasm are difficult to detect without contrast enhancement and fat suppression.

 Caveat: CT with contrast enhancement should *not* be requested except in patients who are too claustrophobic to undergo MRI (since CT is not as sensitive as MRI).

Normal Pressure Hydrocephalus

Presenting Signs and Symptoms

Dementia
Gait disturbance (apraxia of gait)
Urinary incontinence

Common Causes

Previous irritation of the pial surface of the brain due to subarachnoid hemorrhage, diffuse meningitis (postulated to cause scarring of arachnoid villi over brain convexities where CSF absorption usually occurs), or meningeal carcinomatosis

Approach to Diagnostic Imaging

■ 1. Magnetic resonance imaging

- Demonstrates the dilated ventricular system (out of proportion to the degree of sulcal prominence)
- Can exclude the various causes of noncommunicating obstructive hydrocephalus
- Sagittal scans show thinning of the corpus callosum and decreased mamillopontine distance, as well as accentuation of the signal void in the aqueduct of Sylvius and the posterior part of the third ventricle

Note: Distinguishing normal pressure hydrocephalus from neurodegenerative atrophy in the geriatric population is extremely difficult.

■ 2. Radionuclide cisternography

- Demonstrates "reflux" of radionuclide into the lateral ventricles and delayed clearance of isotope from the lateral ventricles and cerebral convexities ("stasis")

Note: This can be a nonspecific finding in older patients with large ventricles and sulci.

Obstructive Hydrocephalus

Presenting Signs and Symptoms

Headache

Nausea, vomiting

Drowsiness

Diplopia, blurred vision

Papilledema

Palsy of the sixth cranial nerve

Pupillary dilatation, coma, decerebrate posturing, abnormal respirations, systemic hypertension, and bradycardia (may develop if increased intracranial pressure is not controlled)

Common Sites of Obstruction and Causes

Foramen of Monro

Neoplasm

Posterior fossa (aqueduct of Sylvius, fourth ventricle, foramen of Luschka, foramen of Magendie)

Congenital stenosis

Neoplasm

Cerebellar infarction/hematoma

Posterior fossa extra-axial and Dandy-Walker cyst

Subarachnoid spaces

Meningitis

Sarcoidosis

Carcinomatosis

Subarachnoid hemorrhage

Other

Venous thrombosis

Choroid plexus papilloma (causes increased CSF production)

Approach to Diagnostic Imaging

■ 1. Magnetic resonance imaging

- Not only demonstrates the dilated ventricular system but may also demonstrate the underlying cause of obstruction to the flow of CSF in the noncommunicating type of hydrocephalus
- Excellent for imaging lesions of the posterior fossa
- Contrast enhancement may assist in distinguishing a congenital posterior fossa cyst from an enhancing cystic neoplasm

Optic Neuritis

Presenting Signs and Symptoms

Visual loss (ranging from a small central or paracentral scotoma to complete blindness) that is usually unilateral

Depressed direct pupillary light reflex

Impairment of color vision

Common Causes

Multiple sclerosis

Viral illness

Ischemia (e.g., temporal arteritis)

Meningitis

Syphilis

Sarcoidosis

Systemic lupus erythematosus

Approach to Diagnostic Imaging

■ 1. Magnetic resonance imaging

- ■ In addition to showing enlargement and contrast enhancement of the optic nerve (also seen on CT), MRI is the preferred study for detecting the characteristic white matter demyelination changes of multiple sclerosis (the most common cause of optic neuritis in adults)

- ■ Fat suppression imaging best visualizes enhancement in the optic nerves

Note: Optic neuritis may be associated with transverse myelitis (Devic's disease).

Orbital Pseudotumor

Presenting Signs and Symptoms

Acute onset of painful proptosis, chemosis, and decreased motility of the extraocular muscles

Usually unilateral (85%) and exquisitely sensitive to steroids

Common Causes

Idiopathic inflammatory reaction (most likely autoimmune, but may be associated with systemic diseases such as Wegener's granulomatosis, lymphoma, fibrosing mediastinitis, thyroiditis, cholangitis, and vasculitis)

Approach to Diagnostic Imaging

■ 1. Computed tomography

- Confusing spectrum of findings includes a discrete soft-tissue mass within the retrobulbar fat and thickening and contrast enhancement of the extraocular muscles, sclera, optic nerve, and lacrimal gland

- MRI is generally used as a problem solver, though some may use it as the primary diagnostic technique

> **Note:** It may be difficult to distinguish orbital pseudotumor from thyroid ophthalmopathy, which (in descending order of severity) involves the inferior, medial, and superior rectus muscles.

Progressive Multifocal Leukoencephalopathy

Presenting Signs and Symptoms

Hemiparesis

Seizures

Blindness

Intellectual dysfunction

Cerebellar or brain stem dysfunction that is relentlessly
progressive

Common Causes

Papovavirus (universal childhood infection that is reac-
tivated in immunosuppressed patients with AIDS,
leukemia, or lymphoma)

Approach to Diagnostic Imaging

■ 1. Magnetic resonance imaging

- Demonstrates asymmetric focal white matter
  lesions in both the cerebrum and cerebellum
  that typically show mild or no mass effect and
  no contrast enhancement (blood–brain barrier
  remains intact)

Note: CT is not as effective in showing this primarily
white matter process.

- Absence of contrast enhancement distinguishes
  PML from abscess and primary CNS lymphoma

Pseudotumor Cerebri (Benign Intracranial Hypertension)

Presenting Signs and Symptoms

Headache and papilledema (increased intracranial pressure) in an otherwise apparently healthy patient

Partial or complete monocular visual loss in 5% (usually intact visual acuity and central visual fields)

Common Causes

Unknown (spontaneous onset and eventual disappearance; patients are often overweight)

In children, may follow withdrawal of steroid therapy or excessive ingestion of vitamin A or tetracycline

Risk Factors

Obesity
Endocrine dysfunction
Sinovenous thrombosis
Hematologic disorders
Increased CSF protein
Meningitis

Approach to Diagnostic Imaging

■ 1. Magnetic resonance imaging or computed tomography

- Excludes a space-occupying mass or venous occlusion causing increased intracranial pressure
- May show associated enlargement of the sella turcica and/or enlargement of the CSF spaces surrounding the optic nerve
- Ventricles are small or normal in size

Radiation Necrosis

Presenting Signs and Symptoms

Progression of neurologic deficit (some patients exhibit no new symptoms)

Onset usually delayed (>6 months) after radiation

Approach to Diagnostic Imaging

■ 1. Magnetic resonance imaging

- Imaging modality of choice for demonstrating both the acute and delayed effects of therapeutic radiation
- Relatively homogeneous, sheet-like increased signal intensity in the radiation field (radiation injury) on T2-weighted sequences
- Heterogeneous and abnormal contrast enhancement may be present (radiation necrosis)

Note: MRI is substantially more sensitive than CT for detecting the predominantly white matter alterations caused by radiation necrosis and radiation injury.

- Proton spectroscopy (no choline peak elevation) may distinguish radiation necrosis from recurrent glioma

■ 2. Positron emission tomography

- In the absence of clinical or radiographic criteria, imaging using ^{18}F-FDG as a marker of cellular metabolism may help distinguish recurrent or residual tumor (hypermetabolic) from areas of radiation necrosis (hypometabolic)

> **Note:** A clear distinction is often difficult because of hypermetabolism that may be seen in radiation necrosis and the common concurrent presence of radiation necrosis and glioma.

9

REPRODUCTIVE

Evis Sala and Hedvig Hricak

FEMALE

▶ SIGNS AND SYMPTOMS

▶ DISORDERS

MALE

▶ **SIGNS AND SYMPTOMS**

▶ **DISORDERS**

Abnormal Uterine Bleeding

Presenting Signs and Symptoms

Excessive menstrual bleeding (menorrhagia)
Nonmenstrual or intermenstrual bleeding (metrorrhagia)
Postmenopausal bleeding

Common Causes

PREMENOPAUSAL

Ovulation (functional ovarian cysts)
Cervicitis
Birth control pills
Anovulatory cycle
Pregnancy
Leiomyoma
Adenomyosis
Malignancy

POSTMENOPAUSAL

Endometrial atrophy
Endometrial polyp
Endometrial hyperplasia
Endometrial cancer

HORMONAL

Vaginal atrophy
Endometrial cancer (about 20% of patients with postmenopausal bleeding)

Approach to Diagnostic Imaging

■ 1. Ultrasound

- Combined transabdominal and transvaginal ultrasound (TVUS) is the preferred initial imaging procedure for detecting abnormalities of the female genital tract

■ 2. Magnetic resonance imaging

- Very useful problem-solving tool (e.g., leiomyoma versus adenomyosis)
- Modality of choice for staging endometrial cancer

Note: See individual sections for recommended workup of specific disorders.

Dysmenorrhea
(Painful Menstruation)

Presenting Sign and Symptom

Pain associated with menses during ovulatory cycles

Common Causes

PRIMARY

No demonstrable lesion affecting the reproductive structures

SECONDARY

Endometriosis
Chronic pelvic inflammatory disease
Cervical stenosis, infection, or neoplasm

Approach to Diagnostic Imaging

■ 1. Ultrasound

- Imaging procedure of choice for detecting or excluding lesions of the female genital tract

Missing Intrauterine Device (IUD)

Presenting Sign and Symptom

Patient unable to feel the attached string (and did not notice that the device was expelled)

Approach to Diagnostic Imaging

■ 1. Ultrasound

- Preferred initial imaging technique if an intrauterine position of the device cannot be confirmed by pelvic examination, uterine sound, or biopsy instrument

■ 2. Magnetic resonance imaging

- IUDs can be safely imaged with MRI, and their presence does not create artifacts that impede image interpretation.

■ 3. Computed tomography

- Can accurately depict the presence of the device within the pelvic cavity.

> **Note:** A plain frontal view is *not* sufficient because it can misdiagnose an extrauterine IUD located in the cul-de-sac.

Infertility

Common Causes

MALE FACTORS (40%)

Deficient spermatogenesis
Varicocele
Cryptorchidism
Retrograde ejaculation into the bladder
Congenital anomalies

FEMALE FACTORS (60%)

Ovulatory dysfunction (20%)
Tubal dysfunction (30%)
Cervical mucus dysfunction (5%)
Other uterine abnormalities (5%)

Approach to Diagnostic Imaging

■ 1. Hysterosalpingography

- ■ Preferred imaging study for demonstrating obstruction of the fallopian tubes (usually secondary to scarring from pelvic inflammatory disease) and uterine synechia (adhesions)

■ 2. Ultrasound or magnetic resonance imaging

- Indicated if the hysterosalpingogram is normal, to detect congenital anomalies of the female genital tract that are seen in up to 10% of women evaluated for infertility or repeated abortion

 Caveat: TVUS cannot always distinguish a submucosal leiomyoma from an endometrial polyp. Sonohysterography has a very high accuracy for detection of endometrial polyps.

Note: Sonohysterography may be used in the evaluation of tubal patency. The identification of free fluid in the pouch of Douglas indicates that at least one fallopian tube is patent.

Chronic Pelvic Pain

Note: Chronic pelvic pain is defined as noncyclic pelvic pain of greater than 6 months duration that is not relieved by strong analgesics.

Causes

GYNECOLOGIC CONDITIONS

Pelvic inflammatory disease
Endometriosis
Leiomyoma
Adenomyosis
Pelvic congestion syndrome

OTHER MEDICAL CONDITIONS

Irritable bowel syndrome
Interstitial cystitis

Approach to Diagnostic Imaging

■ 1. Ultrasound

- Primary imaging technique for the major gynecologic causes

■ 2. Magnetic resonance imaging

- Problem-solving modality (e.g., adenomyosis versus leiomyoma; endometriosis versus dermoid)
- Modality of choice for diagnosis of pelvic congestion syndrome. Three-dimensional T1 gradient-echo sequences performed after the intravenous administration of gadolinium are the most effective for demonstrating pelvic varices.

Congenital Uterine Anomalies

Presenting Signs and Symptoms

Amenorrhea

Infertility, recurrent miscarriages

Intrauterine growth retardation, premature birth

Risk Factors

Intra- and extra-uterine environmental factors such as exposure to ionizing radiation, intrauterine infections, and drugs with teratogenic effects (e.g., thalidomide, DES)

Genetic predisposition

Common Types

Unicornuate uterus

Uterus didelphys

Bicornuate uterus

Septate uterus

Arcuate uterus

Müllerian agenesis or hypoplasia

Vaginal septum

Approach to Diagnostic Imaging

■ 1. Ultrasound

- Preferred initial imaging modality. Sonohysterography provides improved delineation of the endometrium and internal uterine morphology. Three-dimensional US has a higher sensitivity and specificity, with improved delineation of the external uterine contour and uterine volume.

 Caveat: Operator dependent.

■ 2. Magnetic resonance imaging

- MRI is the modality of choice because it has the highest accuracy for evaluation of Müllerian duct anomalies and coexistent secondary diagnoses such as endometriosis and renal anomalies

■ 3. Hysterosalpingography

- Indicated only if US or MRI not available, or if used as the initial test for evaluation of tubal patency in infertile patients

Leiomyoma (Fibroid) of the Uterus

Presenting Signs and Symptoms

Note: Signs and symptoms depend on the location and size of the lesion.

Asymptomatic (detected incidentally on routine pelvic examination or on an imaging study performed for another reason)

Abnormal vaginal bleeding

Pressure symptoms caused by increasing size of the uterus

Acute abdomen (when torsed or undergoing "red" degeneration)

Approach to Diagnostic Imaging

■ 1. Ultrasound

- Preferred initial imaging technique for diagnosing this benign uterine tumor
- Transvaginal studies are helpful for small and submucosal leiomyomas
- Sonohysterography is more accurate than transvaginal US in differentiating submucosal leiomyoma from endometrial polyp

Note: There is no longer any indication for hysterosalpingography in the diagnosis of submucosal leiomyomas.

■ 2. Magnetic resonance imaging

- Indicated if US is negative or inconclusive in differentiating between uterine and adnexal masses or between leiomyoma and adenomyosis, and in searching for submucosal leiomyomas in unexplained bleeding or an infertility workup
- Allows precise determination of size, location, number, and type of degeneration (if present) of leiomyomas, information that is crucial for treatment planning
- MR angiography performed as part of pre-UAE MRI examination can provide useful information on the anatomy of uterine and ovarian arteries (e.g., absent uterine artery, multiple uterine arteries, and ovarian arterial collaterals are associated with lower UAE success rates), as well as the degree of vascularity of a leiomyoma (e.g., hemorrhagic or necrotic leiomyomas usually do not respond to UAE and are best treated by myomectomy or hysterectomy)
- MRI is very useful in monitoring:
  - the effects of hormonal therapy on leiomyomas
  - patients who have undergone myomectomy, as recurrence occurs in up to 15% of patients
  - the success of UAE and assessment of its durability and potential complications, such as intracavitary sloughed leiomyomas, endometritis, and pyometra

---

Note: MRI provides significant advantages over US by accurately mapping the location of the leiomyomas, assessing their perfusion before and after UAE, and allowing definite identification of adenomyosis.

 Caveat: Neither US nor MRI can reliably differentiate benign leiomyoma from the rare malignant leiomyosarcoma.

■ 3. Interventional radiology

- Uterine artery embolization (UAE) can control bulk symptoms in approximately 90% of patients and leads to shrinkage of individual leiomyomas in 48–78% of patients. Subserosal and intramural leiomyomas have a higher UAE failure rate than submucosal leiomyomas.

- MR-guided focused ultrasound thermocoagulation uses MRI to map the leiomyoma in order to deliver thermocoagulation to targeted tissue. This procedure is semi-invasive, obviates the need for ionizing radiation exposure, and has a lower leiomyoma recurrence rate than UAE.

 Caveat: It takes a long time to treat large tissue volumes.

Adenomyosis

Presenting Signs and Symptoms

Menorrhagia and intermenstrual bleeding
Smooth enlargement of the uterus
Nonspecific pelvic pain and bladder and rectal pressure

Approach to Diagnostic Imaging

■ 1. Ultrasound

- TVUS is the recommended initial imaging procedure for demonstrating the heterogeneous
  texture of an enlarged uterus. Real-time imaging
  is crucial.

 Caveat: Many patients with a leiomyomatous
uterus have a similar pattern on US of a diffusely
abnormal uterine texture without evidence of
discrete leiomyomas. When surgery is planned,
distinguishing between leiomyoma and adenomyosis is crucial in patients who wish to preserve
the uterus. Adenomyosis requires hysterectomy
for definitive therapy, whereas leiomyomas can
be treated by selective myomectomy with pres-
ervation of the uterus.

■ 2. Magnetic resonance imaging

- Highly sensitive for detecting adenomyosis and
  accurate in making the critical distinction from
  leiomyoma

Note: CT is *not* applicable in this clinical situation.

Endometrial Polyp

Presenting Signs and Symptoms

Mostly asymptomatic and an incidental finding on TVUS

Postmenopausal bleeding, menorrhagia, intermenstrual bleeding, mucous discharge

Infertility

Risk Factors

More common in patients receiving tamoxifen or on hormone replacement therapy

Approach to Diagnostic Imaging

■ 1. Ultrasound

- TVUS is the modality of choice, with a very high sensitivity and specificity
- Sonohysterography is indicated when there is nonspecific thickening of the endometrium and suboptimal views on TVUS

■ 2. Magnetic resonance imaging

- May be of value in cases when TVUS is inconclusive and biopsy is not possible

Endometrial Hyperplasia

Presenting Signs and Symptoms

Postmenopausal bleeding, menorrhagia, menometrorrhagia

Risk Factors

Unopposed estrogen exposure (chronic anovulatory states, tamoxifen, hormone replacement therapy, estrogen-secreting ovarian tumors) and obesity

Approach to Diagnostic Imaging

■ 1. Ultrasound

- TVUS is the modality of choice, with a very high sensitivity and specificity
- Sonohysterography has the highest accuracy for differentiating hyperplasia from a large endometrial polyp filling the endometrial cavity

■ 2. Magnetic resonance imaging

- May be of value in cases when TVUS is inconclusive and biopsy is not possible

 Caveat: MRI characteristics of endometrial hyperplasia are nonspecific and are similar to those of Stage IA endometrial carcinoma.

Cancer of the Cervix

Presenting Signs and Symptoms

Usually detected by screening Papanicolaou (Pap) test
Vaginal discharge and bleeding (especially after intercourse)

Risk Factors

History of early, frequent coitus and multiple partners
Human papilloma virus infection (type 16 and 18)
Smoking
Immunosuppression

Staging and Treatment Selection

■ 1. Magnetic resonance imaging

- Preferred study for:
  - Demonstrating the tumor
  - Measuring its size
  - Aiding treatment selection by showing direct
    tumor extension to the lower uterine seg-
    ment, vagina, paracervical and parametrial
    tissues, bladder, and rectum
- MRI is superior to CT for preoperative tumor
  visualization and determination of parame-
  trial invasion. However, MRI has significantly
  greater interobserver variability than CT.

■ 2. Computed tomography

- Valuable in advanced disease and in the search for lymph node metastases

 Caveat: Cervical cancer frequently metastasizes to pelvic, inguinal, and retroperitoneal lymph nodes but may not enlarge them. However, both MRI and CT use lymph node enlargement as primary criterion for detecting metastatic involvement.

Note: MRI lymphography using ultrasmall paramagnetic iron particles (USPIO) has shown promising results in significantly improving specificity and maintaining the high sensitivity of conventional MRI.

■ 3. Ultrasound

- TVUS has limited value in the detection of cervical cancer and the determination of stromal invasion or parametrial extension

 Caveat: There is *no* indication for the routine use of excretory urography or barium enema examination (the diagnostic mainstays before cross-sectional imaging).

Treatment Follow-Up

▪ 1. Magnetic resonance imaging

- Modality of choice for monitoring tumor response to radiotherapy as well as evaluating such possible complications as cervical stenosis, fistulae, radiation colitis, and bone marrow changes (ranging from bone marrow edema to insufficiency fracture)
- Study of choice for detecting tumor recurrence within the pelvis

 Caveat: MRI cannot reliably distinguish tumor recurrence from post-radiation changes. Dynamic contrast-enhanced MRI may be helpful in improving specificity and accuracy, but early radiation change continues to pose a problem as it may show contrast-enhancement identical to tumor (up to 6 months following completion of radiotherapy).

▪ 2. Computed tomography

- Valuable in detection of metastatic disease and for guiding percutaneous biopsies

▪ 3. PET/CT

- Useful in the detection of metastatic lymph nodes, with a sensitivity of 91% and a specificity of 100% that are higher than the sensitivity (73%) and specificity (83%) of MRI
- Can be helpful in differentiating tumor recurrence from radiation changes
- Offers added value in patients with recurrent cervical cancer who undergo salvage therapy, as it can provide precise re-staging information.

Cancer of the Endometrium

Presenting Signs and Symptoms

Abnormal uterine bleeding (postmenopausal or recurrent metrorrhagia in a premenopausal woman)

Mucoid or watery vaginal discharge

Predisposing Factors

Delayed menopause

Abnormal menstrual history or infertility

Estrogen-secreting ovarian tumor

Possible Implicated Factors

Obesity

Hypertension

Diabetes mellitus

Breast cancer

Absence of ovulation

Family history of breast or ovarian cancer

Approach to Diagnostic Imaging

■ 1. Ultrasound (TVUS approach preferred)

- Used to measure endometrial thickness in postmenopausal women to select patients suspected of having endometrial carcinoma for dilation and curettage

> **Note:** In a postmenopausal woman not on hormone replacement therapy, an endometrial stripe >5 mm is an indication for endometrial biopsy.

Staging and Treatment Selection

■ 1. Magnetic resonance imaging

- Procedure of choice for demonstrating:
  - Depth of myometrial invasion
  - Extension into the cervix, broad ligaments, parametrium, and ovaries
  - Lymphatic spread to pelvic and retroperitoneal lymph nodes
- Multiphase dynamic contrast-enhanced MRI in sagittal and axial planes is mandatory for high staging accuracy
- MRI lymphography using ultrasmall paramagnetic iron particles (USPIO) has shown promising results for significantly improving specificity and maintaining high sensitivity of conventional MRI

Note: Staging with MRI is superior to that obtained with clinical evaluation and CT.

■ 2. Computed tomography

- Indicated only in advanced cases to search for adjacent organ and pelvic side wall invasion or lymph node metastases

Note: TVUS has been advocated for the assessment of myometrial invasion. However, this method has not been widely accepted because it is subjective, operator-dependent, and significantly inferior to dynamic contrast-enhanced MRI. Furthermore, TUVS is limited in the presence of concomitant uterine pathology (e.g., leiomyoma, adenomyosis). However, 3D US has shown promising results and is under evaluation.

Treatment Follow-Up

■ 1. Magnetic resonance imaging

- MRI is the modality of choice for detection of tumor recurrence within the pelvis. The vaginal vault is the sole site of recurrence in 30–50% of patients; the remainder develop as pelvic or para-aortic lymph node involvement or as systemic spread.

■ 2. Computed tomography

- CT is recommended for evaluation of metastatic disease in the chest and abdomen and for biopsy guidance.

■ 3. PET/CT

- Very useful in surveillance for cancer recurrence and detection of lymph node and distant metastases.

Endometriosis

Presenting Signs and Symptoms

Pelvic pain associated with menses (dysmenorrhea)
Dyspareunia
Pelvic mass
Effect of implants on other organs (e.g., lesions involving large bowel or bladder may cause pain with defecation, abdominal bloating, rectal bleeding with menses, or hematuria and suprapubic pain during urination)

Common Causes

Unknown mechanism for presence of endometrial tissue at ectopic sites outside the uterus (retrograde flow of menstrual bleeding is a hypothesis)

Predisposing Factors

Family history
Delay in childbearing
Müllerian duct anomalies
Asian race

Approach to Diagnostic Imaging

Note: Endometriosis presents as three distinct lesions: ovarian endometrioma, endometrial implants, or adhesions.

 Caveat: Ectopic implants of endometrial tissue generally are too small to be visualized by any imaging method, and laparoscopy is essential to detect and stage endometriosis.

■ 1. Ultrasound

- May demonstrate one or more cystic masses filled with old blood (endometrioma)

> **Note:** Although US can identify the presence of an adnexal lesion, it may be unable to definitively differentiate an endometrioma from other adnexal masses.

■ 2. Magnetic resonance imaging

- Most sensitive modality for diagnosing endometriosis and for differentiating an endometrioma from other adnexal masses, specifically cystic teratomas.

> **Note:** MRI cannot reliably visualize adhesions or intraperitoneal implants. Other imaging modalities (barium enema, CT) may demonstrate the extent of disease (secondary involvement of other organs) but are not sufficiently specific to provide a precise diagnosis.

Cancer of the Ovary

Presenting Signs and Symptoms

Asymptomatic (until very large)
Vague lower abdominal discomfort
Mild digestive complaints
Vaginal bleeding
Late findings include abdominal swelling due to ascites
   and a lobulated or fixed solid mass associated with
   nodular implants in the cul-de-sac

Predisposing Factors

Nulliparity, family history, use of fertility drugs
10% are due to hereditary syndromes such as BRCA-1
   and BRCA-2 mutations (increased risk of breast cancer) and Lynch syndrome II (increased risk of colon
   cancer)

Approach to Diagnostic Imaging

■ 1. Ultrasound

- Preferred initial imaging procedure for demonstrating adnexal tumor, which varies in appearance from a multilocular cyst with vegetations to a complex mass with prominent solid elements

---

> **Note:** Combined gray-scale US and color flow Doppler provides the best lesion characterization.

■ 2. Magnetic resonance imaging or computed tomography

- Indicated when the US findings are inconclusive in determining whether a lesion is benign or malignant

 Caveat: An unequivocal diagnosis of malignancy requires the demonstration of metastases. Nevertheless, even in the absence of metastatic disease, imaging findings can be highly suggestive of malignancy. For example, MRI has a positive predictive value of 92% for determining whether an ovarian tumor is benign or malignant.

Staging and Treatment Selection

■ 1. Computed tomography

- CT is the most commonly performed study for the preoperative staging of suspected ovarian carcinoma. It is particularly useful in evaluating the extent of the disease and thus triaging patients to neo-adjuvant chemotherapy or primary cytoreductive surgery.
- Preferred study for demonstrating:
    - Primary tumor
    - Peritoneal and omental spread
    - Lymphatic metastases to pelvic and retroperitoneal nodes
    - Malignant ascites
    - Hematogenous spread to the liver and lungs

■ 2. Magnetic resonance imaging

- MRI is indicated only if there is a contraindication to the use of iodinated contrast material (e.g., renal failure or allergy) or if the CT findings are inconclusive. MRI requires longer examination time and incurs higher costs than CT.

Note: Contrast-enhanced MRI is the best modality to assess pelvic sidewall invasion and is very sensitive (95%) for detection of peritoneal metastases in the upper abdomen. However, subserosal (bowel) tumor implants are difficult to detect on MRI.

 Caveat: Ovarian carcinoma spreads primarily by peritoneal seeding, with small tumor nodules implanting on the peritoneum, mesentery, and omentum. The role of imaging is to assist surgical planning, determine the surgical expertise required, and diagnose tumor nonresectability.

Treatment Follow-Up

■ 1. Computed tomography

- CT is the modality of choice for treatment follow-up
- Very useful for determining the resectability and extent of recurrent tumor, as well as related complications (e.g., hydronephrosis, bowel obstruction)

■ 2. Magnetic resonance imaging

- MRI is superior to CT in the evaluation of local extent of disease and is the best modality to assess pelvic side wall invasion

■ 3. PET/CT

- Indicated when conventional studies are inconclusive or negative and tumor markers are rising.
- Particularly useful for detecting tumor deposits in mesentery and bowel serosa

 Caveat: Sensitivity in detecting small tumor implants is limited.

Note: US has a limited role in assessment of extent of recurrent tumor and its resectability.

Adnexal/Pelvic Mass (Unspecified)

Presenting Sign and Symptom

Palpable or clinically suspected mass

Approach to Diagnostic Imaging

■ 1. Ultrasound

- Preferred imaging procedure for evaluating patients with a clinically suspected pelvic mass
- Can confirm the presence of a mass, establish its organ of origin, and demonstrate its internal consistency (cystic, complex, or solid)

 Caveat: US is less accurate than CT or MRI for demonstrating tumor extension of a malignant neoplasm or lymph node metastases.

■ 2. Computed tomography

- Preferred imaging method for staging pelvic masses suspected of being malignant on US, especially in the setting of elevated tumor markers
- Superior to US for demonstrating tumor spread to adjacent and distant structures

■ 3. Magnetic resonance imaging

- Problem-solving modality in cases of an indeterminate adnexal mass on US

 Caveat: There is *no* indication for plain abdominal radiographs (too insensitive and nonspecific).

Pelvic Inflammatory Disease

Presenting Signs and Symptoms

ACUTE

Lower abdominal pain, fever, and purulent vaginal discharge that usually begins shortly after menses

CHRONIC

Chronic pain

Menstrual irregularities

Infertility (due to mucosal destruction and tubal obstruction)

Common Sources of Infection

Sexual intercourse

Childbirth (puerperal fever)

Abortion

Note: Patients who use IUDs are particularly susceptible.

Approach to Diagnostic Imaging

Note: In uncomplicated cases that respond well to antibiotic therapy, there is *no* need for imaging studies.

■ 1. Ultrasound

- Demonstrates pyosalpinx or tubo-ovarian abscess complicating pelvic inflammatory disease
- Assesses response to therapy

■ 2. Computed tomography

- May be performed after US to visualize the full extent of disease in severe cases
- Indicated if clinical symptoms mimic appendicitis

Note: MRI is used only if CT is indicated but the patient is allergic to iodinated contrast material. Either US or CT can be used for abscess drainage.

Screening for Prostate Carcinoma

Indications

Screening prostate-specific antigen (PSA) studies and digital rectal examination are recommended for all men annually after age 50 (earlier if positive family history or genetic screening)

If either the screening PSA study or the digital rectal examination is abnormal, proceed directly to US

Clinical Guidelines for Elevated Serum Levels of PSA

>4 ng/mL suggestive of prostate cancer (but can be seen in men with benign prostatic hyperplasia, especially if gland is very large)

Note: Some prostate cancers do not secrete PSA, and thus patients with these tumors do not have elevated PSA levels.

Common Causes

Prostate cancer
Benign prostatic hypertrophy

Approach to Diagnostic Imaging

■ 1. Ultrasound (transrectal)

- Preferred imaging technique for asymptomatic men with an elevated PSA level or abnormal digital rectal examination
- Signs suspicious but nonspecific for malignancy include hypoechoic nodule in the peripheral zone, asymmetric enlargement of the gland with deformation of its contour, and areas of increased vascularity on Doppler study

---

Note: PSA density (ratio of PSA to gland volume) is a helpful indicator of malignancy and can be determined by using US-obtained volume measurements of the gland.

 Caveat: Up to 25% of prostate cancers are isoechoic and indistinguishable from normal parenchyma. In addition, it is difficult for any imaging modality to detect cancer in the midst of benign prostatic hypertrophy (central gland).

- Excellent for guiding systemic needle biopsy, which is often recommended if PSA is elevated and no focal abnormality is detected on digital rectal examination.

Note: Additional imaging studies are not routinely used at present until a diagnosis of prostate cancer is established by biopsy. Combined magnetic resonance and spectroscopic imaging (MRSI) shows promise in localizing prostate cancer for patients with elevated PSA and repeated negative biopsies.

Undescended Testis (Cryptorchidism)

Presenting Signs and Symptoms

Incomplete or improper prenatal descent of one or both testes (occurs in about 3% of newborns; most spontaneously descend, so that by age 1 the incidence is only 1%)

Long-Term Complications (Requiring Orchiopexy)

Infertility due to progressive failure of spermatogenesis
Increased risk of a malignant testicular neoplasm developing (in both the undescended and in the contralateral, normally descended testis)

Approach to Diagnostic Imaging

Note: The use of diagnostic imaging for nonpalpable undescended testes is controversial, with some surgeons preferring to go directly to laparoscopy or operative exploration.

■ 1. Ultrasound

- Sensitive for demonstrating the often atrophic undescended testis if it is located beyond the internal inguinal ring (inguinal canal and spermatic cord)

Note: Identification of the mediastinum testis is important to distinguish an undescended testis from an enlarged lymph node in the area of the cord.

 Caveat: US is of *no* value if the testis is located in the pelvis or abdomen.

■ 2. Computed tomography

- Most valuable for detecting the undescended abdominal testis
- May be useful in postpubertal males or for suspected neoplastic degeneration

 Caveat: CT involves radiation (a consideration in this generally younger age group) and cannot detect an undescended testis smaller than 1 cm.

■ 3. Magnetic resonance imaging

- Preferred approach for detecting undescended testes located at or beyond the internal ring of the inguinal canal, and for demonstrating all complications (especially inflammatory or neoplastic)

Scrotal Pain (Acute)

Common Causes

Testicular torsion (usually in patients younger than age 20; characterized by more acute onset)

Acute epididymo-orchitis (most common after age 20; more gradual onset, often with pyuria)

Vasculitis (e.g., Henoch-Schönlein purpura in children, polyarteritis nodosa in adults)

Trauma

Strangulated, incarcerated hernia

Testicular cancer (10% of testicular cancers present with acute pain)

Approach to Diagnostic Imaging

■ 1. Ultrasound with color Doppler

- Torsion: decreased or absent flow on the symptomatic side
- Epididymo-orchitis: diffuse increase in blood flow on the affected side

■ 2. Radionuclide flow study

- Indicated if ultrasound is equivocal or to evaluate patients with delayed presentation in whom missed testicular torsion is suspected
- Torsion: a rounded cold area surrounded by a rim of increased radionuclide activity reflecting hyperemia (doughnut sign)
- Epididymo-orchitis: a generalized increase in vascular flow to the affected side

Benign Prostatic Hyperplasia (BPH)

Presenting Signs and Symptoms

Varying degrees of bladder outlet obstruction (progressive urinary frequency, urgency, and nocturia due to incomplete emptying and refilling of the bladder)

Decreased size and force of the urinary stream (associated with hesitancy and intermittency)

May have terminal dribbling, almost continuous overflow incontinence, or complete urinary retention

Common Causes

Unknown (may involve hormonal imbalance associated with aging)

Approach to Diagnostic Imaging

Note: BPH is a *clinical* diagnosis. Imaging is indicated to measure the volume of the gland as a determinant in deciding the surgical approach, to follow changes in gland size during medical therapy, and (if needed) to assess the degree of urinary obstruction (residual urine volume). The size of the gland does *not* correlate with the symptoms.

■ 1. Ultrasound

Transrectal

- Demonstrates enlargement and heterogeneity of the gland (specifically the transition zone [central gland])
- Often shows a circumferential surgical pseudo-capsule at the transition zone/peripheral zone interface
- May visualize discrete nodules, as well as nodular thickening of the bladder wall (a sign of long-standing urinary outlet obstruction)

Transabdominal

- Can be used to measure the residual urine volume
- Can evaluate the kidney for the presence of hydronephrosis

Cancer of the Prostate

Presenting Signs and Symptoms

Asymptomatic

May be symptoms of bladder outlet obstruction, ureteral obstruction, hematuria, pyuria (indistinguishable from benign prostatic hyperplasia)

Elevated prostate-specific antigen (PSA)

Localized bone pain (from skeletal metastases)

Elevated serum acid phosphatase (indicating local extension or metastases)

Common Causes

Probably hormone-related

Genetic factors

Approach to Diagnostic Imaging

■ 1. Ultrasound (transrectal)

- Preferred imaging technique once prostate cancer has been suspected by digital rectal examination or an elevated PSA level
- Signs suspicious but not specific for malignancy include hypoechoic nodule (especially in the peripheral zone), mass effect on surrounding tissues, and asymmetric enlargement of the gland with deformation of its contour
- Hypervascularity of tumor on color Doppler
- Permits gland volume measurements necessary for calculating the PSA density (gland volume to PSA ratio)
- Excellent for guiding needle biopsy

Caveat: Up to 25% of prostate cancers are isoechoic and indistinguishable from normal parenchyma.

Note: There is *no* indication for routine MRI in the *pre*-biopsy investigation for prostate cancer. However, the combination of MRI/MRSI may be useful to target biopsy in patients with repeated negative biopsies but PSA levels indicative of cancer.

Staging

■ 1. Magnetic resonance imaging

- The use of combined phased-array and endorectal coils represents the state-of-the-art and most effective imaging technique for assessing local spread (extracapsular extension, seminal vesicle invasion) and metastatic involvement of lymph nodes. The addition of MRSI to MRI significantly improves the specificity of tumor localization.

Note: The inability of MRI (and CT) to detect disease in nonenlarged lymph nodes remains an important limitation. However, MRI lymphography using ultrasmall paramagnetic iron particles (USPIO) has shown promising results that significantly improve the specificity and maintain the high sensitivity of conventional MRI.

 Caveat: MRI/MRSI should be delayed for at least 6–8 weeks after prostate biopsy to avoid under- and/or over-estimation of tumor extent due to the presence of hemorrhage.

■ 2. Computed tomography

- Once considered the "gold standard" for the staging of prostate cancer, but no longer used routinely

Note: CT staging is recommended only if the presence of lymph node metastases is suggested on clinical grounds (markedly abnormal digital rectal examination, PSA >20 ng/mL, Gleason score >8).

■ 3. Radionuclide bone scan

- Single best modality for detecting skeletal metastases (high frequency with prostate cancer)

Note: While at present bone scintigraphy remains the test of choice for the detection of bone metastases, new MR techniques such as whole-body MRI are under evaluation.

 Caveat: Radionuclide bone scan is no longer routinely recommended. It should be ordered only if the PSA exceeds 10 ng/mL or if there are skeletal symptoms.

Treatment Follow-Up

Note: Following primary treatment for prostate cancer, detection of residual or recurrent disease is crucial in order to make prompt treatment decisions for salvage prostatectomy following radiation failure or salvage radiotherapy after radical retropubic prostatectomy (RRP) failure and/or the institution of systemic therapy.

■ 1. Magnetic resonance imaging

- MRI can be used to evaluate both local and systemic recurrence. Endorectal MRI can detect local recurrence even in patients with rising PSA but no palpable mass on digital rectal examination. Endorectal MRI has excellent sensitivity and specificity in the evaluation of local recurrence following RRP.

 Caveat: Following pelvic radiation, however, assessment of intraprostatic tumor location and parameters determining local stage, specifically extracapsular extension and seminal vesicle invasion, may be significantly hindered by tissue changes related to radiotherapy.

■ 2. PET/CT

- Can be useful for treatment monitoring.
- Indicated to evaluate presence of local recurrence as well as recurrent disease in lymph nodes or distant metastases.

 Caveat: PET/CT is most valuable when PSA is greater than 35 ng/mL and/or there was an aggressive Gleason score (≥8) at the time of diagnosis.

Cancer of the Testis

Presenting Signs and Symptoms

Scrotal mass (progressively increasing in size)

Generally painless (pain may be exquisite if hemorrhage into a rapidly expanding tumor occurs; 10% of testicular cancers present with pain)

Often attributed to minor trauma (indicating the time when the mass was first discovered)

Approach to Diagnostic Imaging

■ 1. Ultrasound

- Primary imaging adjunct to physical examination; localizes a mass to the testis and characterizes its internal composition

- Should be obtained if symptoms persist after 10 days of antibiotic therapy

■ 2. Magnetic resonance imaging

- Problem-solving modality performed if US is equivocal, if there is a discrepancy between the physical examination and the US study, if bilateral disease is likely (e.g., lymphoma, leukemia), or as follow-up if a patient has a unilateral testis and an equivocal US study

Staging

■ 1. Computed tomography (abdomen and pelvis)

- Most effective staging procedure for demonstrating the presence and extent of extratesticular spread of tumor (most commonly through the lymphatic system along the gonadal vessels, following the testicular veins to renal hilar nodes on the left or the aortocaval chain on the right, or along the external iliac chain)

> **Note:** Thin-section CT of the lungs is also recommended for early detection of frequent pulmonary metastases. If helical CT is available, scans of the abdomen and pelvis are also often obtained.

■ 2. Magnetic resonance imaging

- Comparable to CT for detecting retroperitoneal lymphadenopathy
- Possible advantages include the ability to distinguish lymph nodes from blood vessels without the use of intravenous contrast material
- Recommended in patients with elevated creatinine, allergy to iodinated contrast material, or retroperitoneal surgical clips (which would degrade the CT image)

> **Note:** If the primary diagnosis is testicular choriocarcinoma, brain MRI should be performed because of the high rate of metastases.

■ 3. PET/CT

- Can be useful for treatment monitoring
- Indicated to evaluate normal-sized lymph nodes detected on CT and/or distant metastases

10

OBSTETRICS

Deborah Levine

Unknown Gestational Age

Common Causes

Inability to recall last menstrual period
Irregular menstrual cycles
Oral contraceptive use

Approach to Diagnostic Imaging

■ 1. Ultrasound

- Preferred imaging technique for estimating gestational age
- Indicated when historical dates are in question or there is a discrepancy between fundal height and dates
- In the *first* trimester, the crown-rump length of the embryo is used to calculate the gestational age
- In the *second* and *third* trimesters, the gestational age and fetal weight are calculated by using measurements of the biparietal diameter of the head, head circumference, abdominal circumference, and femur length
- Nomograms using individual measurements and equations are available to calculate gestational age on the basis of fetal biometry

---

Note: Gestational age calculations are very accurate in the first trimester and become increasingly unreliable closer to term. Therefore, measurements in the third trimester are more appropriately made to assess fetal growth rather than to establish gestational age.

Vaginal Bleeding During Pregnancy

Common Causes
FIRST TRIMESTER

Implantation bleeding (about 10–14 days after fertilization)
Ectopic pregnancy
Spontaneous abortion (threatened, incomplete, or complete)
Intrauterine fetal demise
Molar pregnancy
Marginal subchorionic hematoma

LATE PREGNANCY

Placenta previa
Placental abruption
Preterm labor

Approach to Diagnostic Imaging
■ 1. Ultrasound

- Procedure of choice for demonstrating the obstetrical causes of vaginal bleeding during pregnancy (See individual sections in this chapter.)

Abdominopelvic Pain During Pregnancy

Common Causes

Gallstones
Physiologic hydronephrosis of pregnancy
Urinary tract infection
Renal stones
Fibroid degeneration
Ovarian torsion
Placental abruption
Appendicitis

Approach to Diagnostic Imaging

■ 1. Ultrasound

- Preferred imaging technique for initial assessment of abdominopelvic pain in pregnancy since it has no ionizing radiation and can commonly give a diagnosis. However, if the appendix is not visualized in a patient with right lower quadrant pain and a history suspicious for appendicitis, further imaging is needed.

■ 2. Magnetic resonance imaging

- Indicated if US fails to identify the source of pain (since it also has no ionizing radiation)

■ 3. Computed tomography

- Indicated if US is nondiagnostic and MR is not available, and the pain could be related to a surgical emergency such as appendicitis.

 Caveat: Abdominal and pelvic CT gives a fetal dose of 2–3 rads.

Ectopic Pregnancy

Presenting Signs and Symptoms

Cramping pelvic pain
Spotting (occasionally rapid bleeding leading to shock)
Enlarged uterus but smaller than expected for dates
Possibly tender mass in one adnexa
Lower than expected β-hCG level that does not rise
normally

Predisposing Factors

Pelvic inflammatory disease
Tubal surgery
Endometriosis
Ovulation induction
Previous ectopic pregnancy

Approach to Diagnostic Imaging

■ 1. Ultrasound

- Procedure of choice for demonstrating the extrauterine gestational sac, empty uterus, and secondary signs of ectopic pregnancy
- If US is normal, there is still as much as a 30% risk of an ectopic pregnancy (even if transvaginal technique is used)

Note: When an intrauterine pregnancy is demonstrated by US, the risk of a coexisting ectopic pregnancy is extremely low (about 1 in 17,000–30,000 depending on the patient population). Nevertheless, concurrent intrauterine and ectopic pregnancies do occur, especially in women taking ovulation-inducing drugs.

Early Pregnancy Failure and Embryonic Demise

Presenting Signs and Symptoms

Vaginal bleeding and cramping
Failure of the uterus to grow
Absence of embryonic cardiac activity
Decreasing β-hCG levels

Common Causes

Fetal chromosomal abnormality
Cervical abnormality (incompetent, amputated, lacerated)
Uterine abnormality (leiomyoma, congenital anomaly)
Impaired corpus luteum function
Hypothyroidism
Diabetes mellitus
Chronic renal disease
Infection (especially viruses such as cytomegalovirus, rubella, and herpes)

Approach to Diagnostic Imaging

■ 1. Ultrasound

- Procedure of choice for demonstrating an abnormal gestational sac and/or absence of embryonic cardiac activity
- Commonly used criteria for normal early pregnancy (transvaginal technique):
  - Mean sac diameter 13 mm: yolk sac visible
  - Mean sac diameter 18 mm: embryo visible
  - Embryo length 5 mm (approximately 46 days since LMP): cardiac activity
- Can demonstrate an underlying structural abnormality involving the uterus

---

Note: With endovaginal technique, the absence of cardiac activity in an embryo larger than 5 mm is considered diagnostic of embryonic demise. Embryos smaller than 5 mm without cardiac activity should be rescanned in a few days to confirm demise.

Screening for Chromosomal Abnormalities

Predisposing factors

Family history of chromosomal abnormality

Advanced maternal age (greater than 35 years at time of delivery)

Abnormal serum screening in first or second trimester

Approach to Diagnostic Imaging

First trimester nuchal transluncy performed between 10–14 weeks

- A sagittal high-resolution image of the fetus is taken to measure the lucency behind the neck. This measurement is typically combined with patient age and serum screening to provide a numerical risk (e.g., 1/200 risk) for each of the more common aneuploidies, Trisomy 21, 13, and 18.

Second trimester "genetic sonogram" performed between 16–22 weeks

- This study assesses fetal biometry and anatomy. Specific markers for Trisomy 21 (nuchal thickening, renal dilatation, short humerus, short femur, echogenic bright spot in the heart and other morphologic abnormalities) are given an odds ratio that can be combined with maternal age and serum screening to give a numerical risk of Trisomy 21.

Fetal Presentation and Fetopelvic Disproportion

Presenting Sign and Symptom

Failure of the fetal head to properly descend into the pelvis

Common Causes

Malpositioned fetal head (e.g., breech presentation, hyperextended fetal head, transverse lie)
Small maternal pelvis
Placenta previa
Uterine anomaly or fibroids

Approach to Diagnostic Imaging

■ 1. Ultrasound

- Procedure of choice for determining fetal presentation (fetal part closest to the cervix) and fetal lie (relationship of the long axis of the uterus to the fetus)
- Can distinguish among types of breech presentation when vaginal delivery or version is being considered
  - Frank breech: hips flexed, knees extended (65%)
  - Complete breech: hips flexed, knees flexed (10%)
  - Footling breech: may be associated with umbilical cord prolapse (25%)

■ 2. Magnetic resonance imaging

- Procedure of choice for pelvimetry (usually performed when vaginal delivery is being considered for breech presentation)

Fetal Morphological Abnormalities

Predisposing Factors

Family history of congenital anomalies or genetic illness
Maternal illness or exposure during pregnancy
Substance abuse
Maternal diabetes mellitus that is not in control during
   embryogenesis

Approach to Diagnostic Imaging

■ 1. Level I ultrasound (basic)

- Commonly performed between 17 and 20 weeks
  gestational age
- In addition to fetal measurements and estimates
  of fetal weight and gestational age, the basic
  sonogram includes imaging of the brain,
  heart, outflow tracts, spine, stomach, kidneys,
  urinary bladder, extremities, and umbilical
  cord, placenta, as well as the maternal uterus,
  cervix, and adnexa
- Detects unsuspected fetal anomalies, prompting
  amniocentesis or further imaging

■ 2. Level II ultrasound (targeted or survey)

- Performed when an abnormality is detected during basic US, when there are predisposing factors for fetal anomalies, or when the maternal serum quadruple screen (α-fetoprotein, human chorionic gonadotropin [hCG], Estriol, Inhibin-A) is abnormal
- A detailed evaluation of fetal anatomy, targeted as indicated by the patient's history, is performed by a physician with experience in high-risk obstetric ultrasound

■ 3. Magnetic resonance imaging (fast-sequence)

- Although US remains the primary modality for imaging fetal anomalies, fast-sequence MR imaging can provide additional information in selected cases, particularly for fetal central nervous system abnormalities or if fetal surgery or intervention is planned.

Intrauterine Growth Restriction (IUGR)

Presenting Sign and Symptom

Estimated fetal weight below the 10th percentile for gestational age

Common Causes

Uteroplacental insufficiency

Fetal chromosomal abnormalities

Intrauterine infection (cytomegalovirus, rubella, toxoplasmosis)

Maternal disease (hypertension, preeclampsia, diabetes mellitus, renal disease, malnutrition)

Smoking, alcohol, drug abuse

Approach to Diagnostic Imaging

■ 1. Ultrasound

- Preferred initial imaging study for estimating gestational age and assessing whether fetal growth is proceeding normally
- Can distinguish symmetric from asymmetric IUGR
- *Symmetric* IUGR (the head, abdomen, and femur measurements are all proportionally small) usually occurs early in pregnancy and is commonly associated with chromosome abnormalities or infection
- *Asymmetric* IUGR (the fetal abdomen is disproportionally small relative to the head and femur) usually occurs later in pregnancy and is most often secondary to uteroplacental insufficiency
- Oligohydramnios (markedly decreased amniotic fluid) may be seen in the presence of severe IUGR
- Cord Doppler demonstration of lack or reversal of diastolic flow is an indication for early delivery

Multiple Pregnancy

Presenting Sign and Symptom

Large uterine size for dates

Approach to Diagnostic Imaging

■ 1. Ultrasound

- Demonstrates the presence of multiple embryos or fetuses
- Permits characterization of multiple pregnancies according to the number of amniotic sacs and whether or not the fetuses share a single placenta

---

Note: The relative risk of twin morbidity (prematurity, polyhydramnios, increased incidence of congenital anomalies, discordant growth) is substantially higher if the fetuses share a placenta (monochorionic). Twin-twin transfusion syndrome only occurs if twins are monochorionic. Cord accidents only occur if twins are monoamniotic.

Placental Abruption

Presenting Signs and Symptoms

Vary depending on the degree of placental separation and the extent of blood loss

Third-trimester bleeding (retroplacental hemorrhage that may pass through the cervix and produce vaginal bleeding or be retained behind the placenta)

Severe bleeding may lead to fetal cardiac distress or death and maternal shock

Complications include disseminated intravascular coagulation, acute renal failure, and uteroplacental insufficiency

Risk Factors

Maternal hypertension
Smoking
Cocaine abuse
Autoimmune disorders
Previous history of placental abruption

Approach to Diagnostic Imaging

■ 1. Ultrasound

- Major value is its ability to exclude a placenta previa as the cause of vaginal bleeding
- May often miss the diagnosis of placental abruption due to (1) complete egress of retroplacental blood or (2) isoechogenicity of blood compared with the placenta

Placenta Previa

Presenting Signs and Symptoms

Painless vaginal bleeding (may become massive, bright-red bleeding)

Risk Factors

Previous cesarean section

Uterine abnormality inhibiting normal implantation (fibroid)

Multiple previous pregnancies

Previous placenta previa

Approach to Diagnostic Imaging

■ 1. Ultrasound

- Procedure of choice for demonstrating that part or all of the placenta covers the internal cervical os in a woman in the *third* trimester (most cases of "apparent" placenta previa in the second trimester will "resolve" by the third trimester)

> **Note:** Transperineal (translabial) and transvaginal US may greatly enhance visualization of the cervix, lower uterine segment, and placental edge.

Cervical Incompetence

Presenting Signs and Symptoms

Pelvic pain
Preterm labor

Risk Factors

Prior cervical surgery
DES exposure in utero
Prior cervical incompetence

Approach to Diagnostic Imaging

■ 1. Transvaginal ultrasound

- Procedure of choice for demonstrating the cervical
  length, measured in the longitudinal plane from
  internal to external os

APPENDIX I

■ ■ ■

IMAGING MODALITIES

▶ DIGITAL RADIOGRAPHY (COMPUTED RADIOGRAPHY)

In modern institutions, all radiography, including fluoro-scopically obtained portable images, are now or are rapidly becoming digital. This facilitates increased utilization of Picture Archiving and Communications Systems (PACS), which has transformed radiology from a film-reading spe-cialty to one that is totally filmless, utilizing images read from CRT monitors. This approach is ideally suited to the newer, image-richer, multidetector versions of computed tomography (MDCT), multiple-sequence magnetic reso-nance imaging (MRI), and combined positron emission and computed tomography (PET/CT) systems, making the viewing of large number of images easier by allowing fast displays.

▶ ULTRASOUND (US)

US is the most popular and widely accepted cross-sectional imaging technique in the world. It combines relatively low cost with wide distribution, immediate accessibility, high spatial resolution, and the ability to image in any plane. In this noninvasive modality, high-frequency sound waves produced by electrical stimulation of a specialized crys-tal are passed through the body (reduced in intensity) in relation to the acoustic properties of the tissues through which they travel. The crystal is mounted in a transducer, which also acts as a receiver to record echoes reflected back from the body whenever sound waves strike an interface between two tissues that have different acoustic imped-ance. A water–tissue interface produces strong reflections (echoes), whereas a solid-tissue mass that contains only small differences in composition causes weak reflections. Display of the US image on a television monitor shows both the intensity level of the echoes and the position in the body from which they arose. US images may be dis-played as static gray-scale images or as multiple images that permit movement to be viewed in real time. In general, fluid-filled structures have intense echoes at their borders, no internal echoes, and good through-transmission of the sound waves. Solid structures produce internal echoes of variable intensity.

An additional US technology is the color flow duplex system. In this technique, conventional real-time imaging is combined with Doppler imaging to produce quantitative data and with color to depict motion. The color and intensity represent the direction of flow and the magnitude of the velocity, respectively.

The major advantage of US is its safety. To date, there is no evidence of adverse effects on human tissues at the intensity level currently used for diagnostic procedures. Therefore, US is the modality of choice for examining children and pregnant women, in whom there is potential danger from the radiation exposure of other imaging studies utilizing ionizing radiation. It is an excellent technique for evaluating fetal age, congenital anomalies, and complications of pregnancy.

The major limitation of US is the presence of acoustic barriers, such as air, bone, and barium. For example, air reflects essentially the entire US beam, so that structures beneath it cannot be imaged. This is a special problem in a patient with adynamic ileus and is the major factor precluding US examination of the thorax. Ultrasound also has limited use in very obese patients, a rapidly growing segment of the population in the United States and Western Europe. For an ultrasound study of the pelvis, the patient is usually given large amounts of fluid to fill the bladder, thus displacing the air-filled bowel from the region of interest. In postoperative patients, US may be difficult to perform because of overlying dressings, retention sutures, drains, and open wounds that may prevent the transducer from coming into direct contact with the skin. US is also highly operator-dependent. Extensive technologist (sonographer) and physician (sonologist) training is necessary to produce high-quality images suitable for interpretation.

▶ COMPUTED TOMOGRAPHY (CT)

In this technique, cross-sectional tomographic images are obtained by first scanning a "slice" of tissue from multiple angles with a narrow x-ray beam. Then, relative linear attenuation coefficients (amount of radiation absorbed in tissue) are calculated. These attenuation coefficients are assigned to bytes at a rate of 0.5 MB for every CT image and displayed as a gray-scale image on a CRT monitor. The CT number reflects the attenuation of a specific tissue relative to that of water, which is arbitrarily given a CT number of 0. The highest CT number is that of bone, the lowest that of air. Fat has a CT number of less than 0, whereas soft tissues have CT numbers greater than 0.

The major advantages of CT (especially when enhanced with oral and intravenous iodinated contrast material) over digital radiography are its superb contrast resolution, speed, and the ability to display exquisite anatomic detail in tomographic (MDCT in three-dimensional volumetric) form.

The newest technology in CT is multidetector scanning. In this technique, continual CT scanning is performed as the patient is moved through the gantry containing up to 64 rows of detectors (prototypes of 128 rows-of-detector CTs are already in clinical trials). This permits much faster scanning with substantial reduction of artifacts due to respiratory and cardiac motion. Multidetector CT provides data that can be displayed in three-dimensional images and offers high-quality angiographic studies, including coronary arteriography (of particular value in assessing the patency of coronary bypasses).

Because of its many advantages, CT is now becoming the preferred cross-sectional imaging modality. However, this has raised some questions about the increasing radiation exposure to the patients. Radiation-reducing techniques are being introduced by equipment manufacturers, particularly for pediatric imaging where patient dose is adjusted based on body thickness. The fear of ionizing radiation has led to an increasing use of ultrasound and magnetic resonance imaging, particularly in Western Europe.

▶ MAGNETIC RESONANCE IMAGING (MRI)

This imaging technique basically consists of inducing transitions between energy states by causing certain hydrogen atoms within a powerful static magnetic field to absorb and transfer energy when impacted by a radio pulse of a specific frequency. Various measures of the time required for the material to return to a baseline energy state (relaxation time) can be translated by a complex computer program to a visual image on a CRT monitor. The parameters of the MR image are set by selection of a pulse sequence. Magnets used for MRI are superconducting (cryogenic). For clinical use, they vary in magnetic field strength from 0.5 T to 3 T. Research scanners with 7 T (and even 8 T) magnetic field strength are being tested in several university centers in the United States and Western Europe. Most current clinical MRI scanners in the industrialized world are 1.5 T.

Although the signal intensity of various substances on MR scans is complex and depends on multiple factors, some generalizations can be made:

T1-weighted imaging: Substances causing high (bright) signal intensity include fat, subacute hemorrhage, highly proteinaceous material (e.g., mucus), and slow-flowing blood. Water, as in cerebrospinal fluid or simple cysts, has relatively low signal intensity and appears dark. Soft tissue has an intermediate level of signal.

T2-weighted imaging: Water has a high (bright) signal intensity, whereas muscle and other soft tissues (including fat) tend to have a low signal intensity and appear dark.

Bone, calcium, and air appear very dark on all imaging sequences.

MRI has many of the advantages offered by other imaging modalities, without the associated disadvantages. Like US, MRI does not use ionizing radiation and is capable of directly imaging in multiple planes. Unlike US, MRI depends less on the operator's skill and can penetrate bone and air without a significant decrease in intensity so that the underlying tissue can be clearly imaged. Major advantages of MRI over CT are the far higher soft-tissue contrast resolution, the ability to directly image in any plane, and the use of innumerable different sequences to improve soft-tissue contrast and reduce artifacts.

Although MRI has improved the sensitivity of detecting abnormal tissue, it has had much less effect on specificity. In the head, for example, infarction, edema, tumor, infection, and demyelinating disease all produce identical high signal intensity on T2-weighted images. Other disadvantages of MRI are its high investment cost and operating expenses while an US, for example, can be performed in an office setting. The possibility of patient claustrophobia and the contraindication to imaging in patients with pacemakers and defibrillators (may prevent proper operation) or intracranial ferromagnetic aneurysm clips (may slip and result in hemorrhage) may be patient-related disadvantages of MRI units. New approaches to motion suppression are constantly being developed. Ultrafast techniques for MRI scanning are now available that can provide high spatial resolution images and allow dynamic scanning.

MR angiography (MRA) is a technique that provides high-quality images of the arterial and venous systems with contrast material. Technical refinements and clinical experience are expanding the role of this modality and allow MRA to compete with MDCT in angiography of vascular disease.

MRI has emerged as the imaging modality of choice for evaluating the central nervous system (brain and spinal cord), musculoskeletal system (including joints and spine), pelvis, retroperitoneum, mediastinum, and large vessels. It is equivalent to contrast-enhanced CT for studying focal liver disease and disorders of the spleen, pancreas, and kidneys. It shares with CT the advantages and disadvantages of interpreting possibly neoplastic lymphadenopathy. In specific clinical situations (e.g., most disease processes involving the central nervous system), it is more cost-effective to perform MRI as the initial imaging procedure to achieve a precise diagnosis, rather than obtaining numerous other imaging studies and then having to order an MRI scan anyway.

MRI has also become the problem-solving modality in fetal imaging, because it can provide much more information than ultrasound.

MAGNETIC RESONANCE SPECTROSCOPIC IMAGING (MRSI). MR proton spectroscopic imaging now has two major clinical applications. This modality can be used to stage carcinoma of the prostate by superimposing on the MR image voxels containing data of ratios of normally occurring citrate and choline, which are found to be elevated in cancer. Computer software can assign a color to each voxel where the choline-to-citrate ratio is higher than normal levels. In the post-treatment follow-up of patients with brain tumors, proton spectroscopic imaging can differentiate among recurrent tumor, necrosis, and post-irradiation changes. This approach takes advantage of the fact that normal brain contains N-acetylaspartate. Tumor has a high concentrations of choline, and necrosis gives no signal. In addition, MRSI is emerging as a potentially valuable test for detecting breast cancer.

MAGNETIC SOURCE IMAGING. Magnetic source imaging machines detect tiny magnetic fields created by normally occurring electrical currents in the brain or heart and amplify them using superconducting circuits (SQUIDs), localizing the activity via a mathematical model. The anatomic source of activity is then shown superimposed on a high-resolution MR image, yielding a composite image showing morphology and function. The temporal resolution is real-time. Applications of this technology include localization of seizure activity in patients with epilepsy and identification and localization of focal functional areas in the brain to enable neurosurgeons to avoid these regions during surgical procedures. This modality is also of great value in identifying foci in the heart that are producing life-threatening arrhythmias.

Magnetic source imaging is competing with functional MR imaging (fMRI). Where installed and properly staffed, magnetic source imaging is of special value in planning the preoperative approach to brain tumors.

▶ CONTRAST MEDIA

Various oral and intravenous agents are employed in medical imaging to:

Increase the contrast between different tissues
Depict the hollow viscera
Study blood vessels and the flow within them
Assess organ function
Facilitate interventional procedures

Contrast media are widely used with all imaging modalities except US (although even in this area vascular applications have been developed and have proven to be valuable). They are not routinely employed because their use significantly increases the price of the procedure.

BARIUM SULFATE. This inert material is used as a suspension in water primarily to study the gastrointestinal tract. Suspension agents are employed to prevent sedimentation and flocculation. Double-contrast techniques using air (or methylcellulose in enteroclysis) provide superb depiction of mucosal-surface detail.

WATER-SOLUBLE, IODINATED CONTRAST MEDIA. These chemicals can directly visualize the blood vessels (arteriography, venography) or opacify the urinary tract after being excreted by the kidneys. The use of low osmolar or nonionic contrast materials reduces the risk of minor complications and the painful and unpleasant symptoms that may commonly follow the injection of hypertonic iodine-containing contrast media. They are also apparently safer than the hyperosmolar contrast agents and have a lower incidence of severe reactions.

Water-soluble contrast media are now most frequently used to increase contrast resolution in CT scanning. They can indicate whether an area of abnormality has increased or decreased vascularity, compared with adjacent normal tissue. In the brain, contrast enhancement implies that there has been a break in the blood–brain barrier.

Water-soluble contrast materials are used in routine radiography to demonstrate fistulas, sinuses, anastomotic post-operative leaks, and perforations. As an enema, they are used to evaluate suspected colonic perforation and post-operative anastomotic leaks, as well as to soften hard stool in patients with severe constipation.

ULTRASOUND CONTRAST AGENTS. Contrast agents are now available to increase the sensitivity of both US and Doppler studies, as well as to enhance the signal intensity and to widen the applications of these procedures. Most US contrast agents are based on stabilized gas microbubbles. Intravenously injected stabilized gas bubbles must be less than 5 µm in diameter to pass through the pulmonary capillaries. For some contrast media, high-frequency harmonic waves are reflected from the surface of the microbubbles, and if the instrument is tuned to only receive harmonic frequencies, signals from tissues surrounding the vessels can be eliminated.

Another approach for US contrast media is the use of perfluorochemicals, which are inert, dense fluids that can be used in emulsions and are highly US reflective. They are eliminated from the blood stream by phagocytosis, making the liver and spleen visible, or by evaporation through the lungs.

US contrast media are used to enhance visualization of vessels in tumors, to demonstrate vessel stenoses, to study heart disease, and even to perform US hysterosalpingography.

MAGNETIC RESONANCE CONTRAST AGENTS. At present, intravascular, extracellular chelates of gadolinium are used as tissue-enhancing agents to produce effects similar to those of iodinated contrast media in CT. They permit diagnoses that otherwise would require long T2-weighted images to be made on shorter T1-weighted sequences, thus reducing motion artifact. MR contrast agents are far safer than even the nonionic iodinated compounds used in conventional radiography and CT.

Specific contrast agents for the liver, using minute iron oxide particles that are captured by the reticuloendothelial system and give an extremely low-intensity signal, have been approved by the FDA and are slowly receiving acceptance despite their high cost.

There is a substantial need for an orally administered MR contrast medium to outline the gastrointestinal tract. Currently, contrast media consisting of water-containing, hyperosmolar additives (to attract extra-cellular fluid) promise to become the best way to opacify the bowel. Water can be an either high- or low-intensity contrast medium, depending on the imaging sequence used.

▶ NUCLEAR MEDICINE INSTRUMENTATION

SCINTILLATION CAMERA (ANGER CAMERA). This instrument consists of one, two, or three large, flat, rectangular sodium iodide crystals up to 50 cm in length and 40 cm in width. Photons from the radioactive tracer produce luminescence in the crystal, which is then augmented by 5–7 times by a large number of arrayed photo-multiplier tubes. The two-dimensional location of the source of the signal, which is determined by computing the relative intensity of luminescence emitted by the multiple photomultiplier tubes, is displayed on an oscilloscope and then recorded on film.

▶ SINGLE PHOTON EMISSION TOMOGRAPHY (SPECT)

In this technique, the detector system rotates around the patient. The signal from the radioactive sources within the body is acquired from multiple projections and integrated using a computer algorithm somewhat similar to but more complicated than that used for CT.

▶ POSITRON EMISSION TOMOGRAPHY (PET)

Positron-emitting materials such as radioactive carbon (^{10}C, ^{15}C) or oxygen (^{15}O) have fewer neutrons than protons. They are produced in generators or cyclotrons by bombardment of atoms with protons or deuterons. Many are extremely short-lived. When a positron-emitting isotope is introduced into the body, it enters into annihilation reactions with electrons to produce a pair of gamma photons (each with an energy of 511 keV). These gamma photons radiate linearly in opposite directions at an angle of 180°. When they excite opposing detectors circling around the patient, the signals are transformed into an image using an algorithm similar to that used in CT.

Today, PET is primarily employed in the search for metastases when CT or MRI is inconclusive. Clinical scanning is predominantly performed with fluorodeoxyglucose tagged with fluorine 18 (^{18}F-FDG). Studies to determine the viability of myocardium following heart attacks are also performed, but not as frequently. PET is also used in functional imaging to identify foci initiating epileptic seizures and to aid in diagnosing Alzheimer's disease.

The disadvantages of PET are its relatively poor spatial resolution (which is improving) and its high cost (which is reducing with increasing use of this modality).

PET/CT. PET/CT, a hybrid modality based on the mechanical fusion of PET and CT systems in the same scanner, is rapidly gaining acceptance. It has totally superceded PET alone, providing excellent localization for the PET signal by utilizing internally registered CT images and thus overcoming the previous lack of good spatial resolution of this modality. The fusion of PET and CT also reduces the time of the procedure since rod source based transmission images (needed for localization in stand-alone PET units) are no longer needed in combined scanners.

APPENDIX II

■ ■ ■

RELATIVE COSTS OF IMAGING PROCEDURES

Medical imaging has become an indispensable tool in the practice of modern medicine. New and continually improving sophisticated imaging modalities, as well as hybrid imaging such as MR spectroscopy and PET/CT and initial experience with PET/MRI, have permitted more specific diagnoses and better therapeutic approaches, while also significantly increasing the cost of healthcare. Conversely, the widespread availability of diagnostic imaging has contributed to transforming medical care into a lower-cost, predominantly outpatient activity. This has permitted hospital stays to become shorter or even to be eliminated, as well as improvements in longevity and quality of life. Nevertheless, improvements in patient care have come at a substantial cost. In 2006, health care expenditures in the United States were well over two trillion dollars, representing more than 16% of the Gross Domestic Product (GDP).

With the ever-escalating cost of medicine, it is important to be constantly aware of the patient charges for different tests and procedures ordered. Knowing the price of these studies could lead to a reduction in unwarranted and duplicated examinations and serve as an impetus to decreasing health care costs through a well-reasoned approach to diagnostic imaging.

A single costly study that gives precise information and eliminates the need for further imaging is generally the soundest approach. It is important to realize that adding the expense of a more elaborate and expensive test to a relatively inexpensive one will cost the patient (payer) more than if the more sophisticated procedure had simply been ordered and performed initially.

Over the past few years, the price of standard radiographic examinations has generally risen at a rate commensurate with inflation. The dramatic increase in the cost of medical imaging has reflected technological advances in cross-sectional imaging and the conversion to a digital infrastructure (Picture Archiving and Computerized Systems: PACS) that has eliminated analog and hard copy imaging.

Because charges vary widely among various institutions and in different geographic regions, the relative costs (technical and professional) listed below are expressed as multiples of the plain frontal and lateral radiographic examination of the chest, which is designated as "x."

Barium enema	2.5x
Upper gastrointestinal series	3x
Excretory urogram	3x
Hysterosalpingogram	3x
Ultrasound	3x
Radionuclide scan (lung, bone)	3–4x
Echocardiogram	4–5x
CT	7–10x
MRI	8–12x
Angiography	8–12x
MR spectroscopic imaging	10–14x
PET/CT	26x

There has been no real change in the ratio of the cost of CT and MRI relative to the simpler radiographic procedures that were the standard of yesteryear. However, what has changed is that CT has become the standard and basic imaging procedure for the abdomen and even for the chest. It has virtually replaced the less expensive excretory urogram and even supplanted many ultrasound examinations. MRI has become the major problem solving modality, except in the musculoskeletal system and pelvis, where it is often the basic imaging approach. The impact on cost is exacerbated by the addition of PET/CT, which is becoming the accepted procedure for detecting metastatic lymph nodes and the spread of many cancers, though at a cost more than 25 times that of plain chest radiographs. In summary, the increased precision and accuracy of modern imaging, which has so positively influenced medicine, does have a concomitant cost.

Therefore, it is critical that the internist, family physician, and other clinicians who order imaging studies become aware of the advantages of the various radiological procedures and their proper sequencing in order to obtain a precise diagnosis, to guide therapy, and to follow its aftermath. By following the suggestions outlined in this book and not duplicating examinations, it will be possible to enhance patient care while limiting costs as much as possible.

APPENDIX III

CONTRAST REACTION

Part I

■ ■ ■ ────────────────────────────

Preventing Contrast-Induced Injury: Iodinated Contrast

Daniel Brewer

Contrast-Induced Nephropathy (CIN)

Presenting Signs and Symptoms

Contrast-induced nephropathy (CIN) is defined as an increase in serum creatinine of >25% of baseline value following the intravascular administration of contrast material without alternative explanation.

Risk Factors

Chronic renal disease

The estimated glomerular filtration rate (eGFR) is typically calculated on the basis of serum creatinine, age, weight, and gender. It can also be calculated on the basis of a 24 h urine collection.

- CIN is rare in patients with an eGFR >60 mL/min
- Those with an eGFR between 30 and 60 mL/min are at moderate risk
- Those with an eGFR below 30 mL/min are at high risk

Diabetes mellitus
Congestive heart failure

Sepsis or acute hypotension
Dehydration
Age >70 years
Previous chemotherapy
Organ transplantation
Other nephrotoxic drugs
  Loop diuretics, aminoglycosides, vancomycin, NSAIDs,
    amphotericin B
HIV or AIDS

Preventive Strategies

■ 1. Avoidance of other nephrotoxic agents

- If possible, NSAIDs, diuretics, and other nephro-toxic drugs should be held for 48 h prior to the study.

■ 2. Fluid administration

- Volume loading (orally as an outpatient, intrave-nously as an inpatient) prior to the administra-tion of contrast material reduces the risk of CIN
- This must be balanced against the risk of volume overload, especially in patients with congestive heart failure. Volume loading is not indicated in patients on dialysis.
- A typical hydration regimen is 0.9% NaCl at 1 mL/kg/h for 12 h prior to the procedure and for 12 h afterward.

■ 3. Minimizing contrast administration

- The risk of CIN increases with the volume of con-trast material, and if a second dose of contrast is given within 72 h.

■ 4. Choice of contrast material

- Low-osmolar contrast medium is associated with a lower incidence of CIN. There is controversy about differences among low-osmolar agents.

■ 5. Pharmacologic prophylaxis

- Acetylcysteine (Mucomyst®) given prior to contrast studies may reduce the incidence of CIN.

■ 6. Metformin

- Metformin does not cause CIN, but the adverse effects of Metformin are more likely to occur in the setting of CIN. Therefore, most authorities recommend holding Metformin for 48h after a contrast study and reinstituting it only after renal function has been re-evaluated with a serum creatinine. Patients with an eGFR <60mL/min might also be considered for holding Metformin 24 or 48h prior to the study.

Follow Up

Any patient at high risk (eGFR <30mL/min) should have a followup serum creatinine 48h after contrast material has been administered.

Part II

■ ■ ■

Preventing Contrast-Induced Injury: Gadolinium

N. Reed Dunnick

Nephrogenic Systemic Fibrosis

Presenting Signs and Symptoms

Nephrogenic systemic fibrosis (NSF) is a systemic fibrosing disorder that has been found in patients with chronic renal disease. Patients may present with erythematous and indurated plaques of the skin, primarily in the extremities. It may result in flexion contractures, pain, paresthesias or pruritus. It is a systemic disorder that may involve other organs resulting in variable end-organ damage and even death.

Risk Factors

Chronic renal disease

The estimated glomerular filtration rate (eGFR) is typically calculated on the basis of serum creatinine, age, weight, and gender. It can also be calculated on the basis of a 24 h urine collection.

- NSF is rare in patients with an eGFR >60 mL/min
- Those with an eGFR between 30 and 60 mL/min are at moderate risk
- Those with an eGFR below 30 mL/min are at high risk

Hepatorenal syndrome
Perioperative liver transplantation
Liver failure

Preventive Strategies

■ 1. Avoidance of gadolinium-based contrast agents

- The use of a gadolinium-based contrast agent should be avoided unless the diagnostic information is essential and not available through other imaging studies.

■ 2. Minimizing contrast administration

- When administering a gadolinium-based contrast agent, the recommended dose should not be exceeded and a sufficient period of time for elimination of the agent from the body should be allowed prior to any readministration.

■ 3. Dialysis

- Dialysis treatment should occur ideally within 3 h after the administration of the gadolinium-based contrast material. A second dialysis session may be performed within 24 h if indicated.
- Patients undergoing peritoneal dialysis should have no periods with a dry abdomen in which the peritoneal cavity contains no dialysate.

Bibliography

Broome DR, Girguis MS, Baron PW, Cottrell AC, Kjellin I, Kirk GA. Gadodiamide-associated nephrogenic systemic fibrosis: Why radiologists should be concerned. American Journal of Roentgenology 188:586–592, 2007.

Kuo PH, Kanal E, Abu-Alfa AK, Cowper SE. Gadolinium-based MR contrast agents and nephrogenic systemic fibrosis. Radiology 242:647–649, 2007.

Sadowski EA, Bennett LK, Chan MR, Wentland AL, Garrett AL, Garrett RW, Djamali A. Nephrogenic systemic fibrosis: Risk factors and incidence estimation. Radiology 243:148–157, 2007.

Subject Index

Printed in the United States